CHINESE QIGONG MASSAGE

-General Massage-

Dr. Yang Jwing-Ming

DISCLAIMER

The author(s) and publisher of this material are not responsible in any manner whatsoever for any injury which may occur through reading or following the instructions in this material.

The activities, physical or otherwise, described in this material may be too strenuous or dangerous for some people, and the reader(s) should consult a physician before engaging in them.

Publisher's Cataloging in Publication
(Prepared by Quality Books Inc.)

Yang, Jwing-ming.
   Chinese qigong massage : general massage / Jwing-ming Yang.
   p. cm.
   Includes bibliographical references and index.
   ISBN 0-940871-25-4(pbk.)
   ISBN 0-940871-26-2(cloth)

   1. Massage--China. 2. Ch'i kung. 3. Massage--China--History.
I. Title. II. Title: Ch'i kung massage.

RM721.C5   615.822
                                        QBI91-1573

Second Printing 1994
10,3

ISBN: 0-940871-25-4

Printed in USA

YMAA Publication Center
Yang's Martial Arts Association (YMAA) 楊氏武藝協會

38 Hyde Park Avenue • Jamaica Plain, Massachusetts 02130

氣

魯城曲阜姜建業

Dedicated to my wife
Mei-Ling Yang
and my children
James C. Yang
Kathy K. Yang
Nicholas C. Yang

ACKNOWLEDGMENTS

Thanks to A. Reza Farman-Farmaian for the photography, Wen-Ching Wu for the drawings, Michael Wiederhold for the typesetting, and Douglas Goodman for his drawings and cover design. Thanks also to John Chris Belskis for general help, to David Ripianzi, James O'Leary, Jeffrey Pratt, Jenifer Menefee, and many other YMAA members for proofing the manuscript and for contributing many valuable suggestions and discussions. Special thanks to Alan Dougall for his editing and to Mr. Jianye Jiang for his beautiful calligraphy. Again, deepest appreciation to Dr. Thomas G. Gutheil for his continued support.

ABOUT THE AUTHOR

Dr. Yang Jwing-Ming was born on August 11th, 1946, in Xinzhu Xian, Taiwan, Republic of China. He started his Wushu (Gongfu or Kung Fu) training at the age of fifteen under the Shaolin White Crane (Bai He) Master Cheng Gin-Gsao. Master Cheng originally learned Taizuquan from his grandfather when he was a child. When he was fifteen years old, he started learning White Crane from Master Jin Shao-Feng, and he followed him for twenty-three years until Master Jin's death.

In thirteen years of study (1961-1974) under Master Cheng, Dr. Yang became an expert in the White Crane style of Chinese martial arts, which includes both the use of barehands and of various weapons such as saber, staff, spear, trident, two short rods, and many other weapons. With the same master he also studied White Crane Qin Na (or Chin Na), Tui Na and Dian Xue massages, and herbal treatment.

At the age of sixteen, Dr. Yang began the study of Taijiquan (Yang Style) under Master Kao Tao. After learning from Master Kao, Dr. Yang continued his study and research of Taijiquan with several masters and senior practitioners such as Master Li Mao-Ching and Mr. Wilson Chen in Taipei. Master Li learned his Taijiquan from the well-known Master Han Ching-Tan, and Mr. Chen learned his Taijiquan from Master Chang Xiang-San. Dr. Yang has mastered the Taiji barehand sequence, pushing hands, the two-man fighting sequence, Taiji sword, Taiji saber, and Taiji Qigong.

When Dr. Yang was eighteen years old he entered Tamkang College in Taipei Xian to study Physics. In college he began the study of traditional Shaolin Long Fist (Changquan or Chang Chuan) with Master Li Mao-Ching at the Tamkang College Guoshu Club (1964-1968), and eventually became an assistant instructor under Master Li. In 1971 he completed his M.S. degree in Physics at the National Taiwan University, and then served in the Chinese Air Force from 1971 to 1972. In the service, Dr. Yang taught Physics at the Junior Academy of the Chinese Air Force while also teaching Wushu. After being honorably discharged in 1972, he returned to

Tamkang College to teach Physics and resume study under Master Li Mao-Ching. From Master Li, Dr. Yang learned Northern style Wushu, which includes both barehand (especially kicking) techniques and numerous weapons.

In 1974, Dr. Yang came to the United States to study Mechanical Engineering at Purdue University. At the request of a few students, Dr. Yang began to teach Gongfu (Kung Fu), which resulted in the foundation of the Purdue University Chinese Kung Fu Research Club in the spring of 1975. While at Purdue, Dr. Yang also taught college-credited courses in Taijiquan. In May of 1978 he was awarded a Ph.D. in Mechanical Engineering by Purdue.

In 1980, Dr. Yang moved to Houston to work for Texas Instruments. While in Houston he founded Yang's Shaolin Kung Fu Academy, which was taken over by his student Mr. Jeffery Bolt after he moved to Boston in 1982. Dr. Yang founded Yang's Martial Arts Academy (YMAA) in Boston on October 1, 1982.

In January of 1984 he gave up his engineering career to devote more time to research, writing, and teaching. In March of 1986 he purchased property in the Jamaica Plain area of Boston to be used as the headquarters of the new organization, Yang's Martial Arts Association. The organization has continued to expand, and, as of July 1st 1989, YMAA has become just one division of Yang's Oriental Arts Association, Inc. (YOAA, Inc.).

In summary, Dr. Yang has been involved in Chinese Wushu since 1961. During this time, he has spent thirteen years learning Shaolin White Crane (Bai He), Shaolin Long Fist (Changquan), and Taijiquan. Dr. Yang has more than twenty years of instructional experience: seven years in Taiwan, five years at Purdue University, two years in Houston, Texas, and since 1982 in Boston, Massachusetts.

In addition, Dr. Yang has also been invited to offer seminars around the world to share his knowledge of Chinese martial arts and Qigong. The countries he has visited include Canada, Mexico, France, Italy, Poland, England, Ireland, Switzerland, and Germany.

Dr. Yang has authored fifteen other volumes on the martial arts and Qigong:

1. Shaolin Chin Na; Unique Publications, Inc., 1980.
2. Shaolin Long Fist Kung Fu; Unique Publications, Inc., 1981.
3. Yang Style Tai Chi Chuan; Unique Publications, Inc., 1981.
4. Introduction to Ancient Chinese Weapons; Unique Publications, Inc., 1985.
5. Chi Kung - Health and Martial Arts; Yang's Martial Arts Association (YMAA), 1985.
6. Northern Shaolin Sword; Yang's Martial Arts Association (YMAA), 1985.
7. Advanced Yang Style Tai Chi Chuan, Vol.1, Tai Chi Theory and Tai Chi Jing; Yang's Martial Arts Association (YMAA), 1986.
8. Advanced Yang Style Tai Chi Chuan, Vol.2, Martial

Applications; Yang's Martial Arts Association (YMAA), 1986.

9. Analysis of Shaolin Chin Na; Yang's Martial Arts Association (YMAA), 1987.
10. The Eight Pieces of Brocade; Yang's Martial Arts Association (YMAA), 1988.
11. The Root of Chinese Chi Kung - The Secrets of Chi Kung Training; YMAA Publication Center, 1989.
12. Muscle/Tendon Changing and Marrow/Brain Washing Chi Kung - The Secret of Youth; YMAA Publication Center, 1989.
13. Hsing Yi Chuan - Theory and Applications; YMAA Publication Center, 1990.
14. The Essence of Tai Chi Chi Kung - Health and Martial Arts; YMAA Publication Center, 1990.
15. Qigong for Arthritis; YMAA Publication Center, 1991.

Dr. Yang has also produced the following videotapes:

1. Yang Style Tai Chi Chuan and Its Applications; Yang's Martial Arts Association (YMAA), 1984.
2. Shaolin Long Fist Kung Fu - Lien Bu Chuan and Its Applications; Yang's Martial Arts Association (YMAA), 1985.
3. Shaolin Long Fist Kung Fu - Gung Li Chuan and Its Applications; Yang's Martial Arts Association (YMAA), 1986.
4. Shaolin Chin Na; Yang's Martial Arts Association (YMAA), 1987.
5. Wai Dan Chi Kung, Vol. 1 - The Eight Pieces of Brocade; Yang's Martial Arts Association (YMAA), 1987.
6. Chi Kung for Tai Chi Chuan; YMAA Publication Center, 1990.
7. Qigong for Arthritis; YMAA Publication Center, 1991.

Dr. Yang Jwing-Ming

FOREWORD

Dr. Wu Chengde
Houston Institute of Chinese
Martial Arts and Medicine

Traditional Chinese medicine developed out of the experiences accumulated over thousands of years in the battle against disease. It has helped more than a billion Chinese to both maintain their health and prevent illness. Qigong massage has a long history, and has been an important part of Chinese medical system. Chinese Qigong massage, like other Chinese medical practices, is considered an important and effective method of treating and even preventing disease. For thousands of years it has had an important role in Chinese medicine.

The theory of Qigong massage, like other Chinese medical practices, has been built on the foundation of the concept of "Qi." It especially emphasizes the smooth circulation of Qi, its proper level, the quality of its circulation, and also how to use it to prevent disease. In fact, compared with other forms of Chinese medicine, Qigong massage has its own unique effectiveness and benefits. It is therefore commonly used together with Chinese herbs and acupuncture to provide a treatment which is more effective than would be possible with any one form of treatment alone.

The advantages of practicing Qigong are that it does not require a large space or any equipment, and it is easy to learn and practice. Qigong massage can be used anywhere and anytime.

For the last several decades I have been engaged in study, research, and treatments related to the Chinese martial arts and traditional medicine. In addition to filling demanding jobs as a professor at the Shanghai Chinese Medical Institute and as Head Physician at Longhua Hospital, I was also appointed Bone Injury Category Educational Minister of the Chinese Medical Association in China, Administrator of the Shanghai Chinese Medical Study Society, Vice Minister of the Injury Category Study Society, member and Research Administrator of the Shanghai Recovery Medical Study Society, member of the Chinese Shanghai Athletic Medical Society, member of the Chinese Wushu Study Association, and also advisor of the Yangtze River Wugong Medical Treatment Research Institute. I have therefore had countless chances to work with many other medical experts.

In 1989, before I was invited to Houston and later took up residence here, I was already very interested in investigating the position of Chinese medicine in America. Because Chinese medicine is a treasure to human health and happiness, and has been built on the foundation of the relationship of Qi to man's physical and mental bodies, over the course of several thousand years of study and research its experiences and achievements are in some ways very different from those obtained by Western medicine.

In the last two years, I was very surprised to discover that almost every American praises and favors Chinese cooking and says, "Chinese food tastes good." However, only a very few of them know anything about Chinese medicine and its achievements. Chinese medicine in America is still in its infancy. Because of the cultural differences between West and East, people can easily become confused about the concepts of Chinese medicine. This is especially true since science today still cannot understand and accept the concept of "Qi," or study it objectively. Under these conditions, it is especially necessary and urgent for knowledgeable, experienced Qigong researchers, when they publish articles or books, to maintain a centered and neutral viewpoint in their discussions. Only then can confusion be avoided and the general public be encouraged to get involved.

After I came to the United States, I was very fortunate to meet Dr. Yang Jwing-Ming and to learn that Dr. Yang has a deep understanding of both Chinese martial arts and Qigong. His publications are numerous and profound. His dream is to greatly increase the exchange of culture between East and West. He believes, therefore, that it is his responsibility to help introduce Chinese culture to the West, especially Wushu and medical Qigong.

In Dr. Yang's sincerely written works, the reader discovers clear explanations based on his scientific background. His approach of using the scientific method to explain the traditional experience is accurate and objective. Therefore, I am very happy to write the foreword for this book, "Chinese Qigong Massage." This will also fulfill part of my wish to help in the development of Chinese culture in Western society.

吴诚德

Dr. Wu Chengde
September, 1991

FOREWORD

Dr. Yang Jwing-Ming, Ph.D.

Although modern medicine has brought us healthier lives and has significantly extended the average lifespan, there are still many problems that it does not know how to deal with. Modern medicine will often cure one symptom, only to create another. Many treatments seem to be designed only to provide relief from symptoms, rather than identifying and treating the root of the problem.

Even though today's medicine has reached a higher level than ever before, if we compare it to the medicine that we will have in another hundred or a thousand years, it is clear that medicine is only in its infancy.

When looked at objectively, it is clear that there are still many problems with Western medicine. First, the research of the past 50 years has focused on curing, and has virtually ignored prevention. This means that the whole attention of the medical establishment has been focused on treating problems after they have manifested. Attention is given to educating the public only when a situation has become serious. The medical knowledge or medical common sense of the general public is still at the primary school stage.

Another problem with Western medicine is that it concentrates solely on the physical problem and ignores inner energy (bioelectricity or Qi). Few Western physicians understand that Qi is at the root of every sickness, and is the source of the failure of any physical organ or cell. If you wish to prevent sickness, your first concern must be the Qi which is circulating in the body. If there is a persistent abnormality in the supply or circulation of Qi, the physical body will be damaged and symptoms will manifest. If we wish to cure the root of a sickness, we must first resolve any problems with the Qi. If we regulate the Qi supply and circulation back to normal, we can repair the physical damage and regain health. In light of this, it would seem that the best course for future medical research would be to determine the role Qi plays in our health.

Because Western medicine is unfamiliar with Qi, it has been unable to deal with the mental illnesses which are related to energy imbalances in the brain. It is also totally unprepared to deal with the spiritual side of the human body. According to Chinese Qigong and medical science, the human spirit is closely related to the mind and the Qi which is circulating through the brain.

In less than a century, science has made great strides in physical medicine, however, it has failed almost completely to investigate our internal energy. Because of this, modern medicine has been only half successful.

Science has recently discovered that the growth hormone can slow down the aging process. For many centuries, an important part of Chinese Qigong practice has been learning how to use the mind to lead Qi to the pituitary gland in the brain in order to reactivate and maintain the production of the growth hormone. Although it was not understood precisely how this occurred in the body, nourishing the brain with Qi proved to be an effective way to increase the lifespan.

I believe that if East and West can sincerely work at exchanging knowledge, humanity can have a bright and healthy future. During the next fifty years we must study the mental and spiritual sides of medicine which are related to Qi. Our understanding of medicine will be complete only when we understand this invisible side of our beings. The various institutions that are engaged in medical research should begin allocating money and effort to this field now. Those that do will be considered the pioneers of the medicine of the future.

PREFACE

The Chinese people have always believed that in order to have harmony, two universal forces must be in balance. These two forces are classified as Yin (negative) and Yang (positive). When these Yin and Yang forces interact, Qi (energy) is produced and life is generated. This close relationship between life and Yin and Yang is the way of "Dao" (or Tao). The theory of Yin and Yang has given birth to a large part of Chinese culture, and has had a particularly great influence on Chinese medicine and Qigong.

It is believed that in order to have a long, healthy, and happy life, you have to balance the Yin and Yang in your body. Traditionally, the Qi body (internal energy body) is considered to be the Yin body, while the physical body is the Yang body. While the physical body can be seen, the Yin body cannot be seen, it can only be felt. Yin energy is the origin of life and makes possible the growth of Yang. Therefore, when Yin energy weakens or suddenly increases, the result will be manifested in the Yang (physical) body. If the imbalance persists, physical damage or even failure to function will occur in the body.

For this reason, practitioners of Chinese medicine and Qigong have always devoted a major part of their practice and research to maintaining the balance of Yin and Yang. In addition to developing physical exercises to maintain the health of the physical body, they have also been concerned with maintaining an abundant supply of Qi and keeping it circulating smoothly.

In the last fifteen years, Qi theory has gradually been accepted by Western physicians. It is now believed that Qi is what has come to be called "bioelectricity." It is the (Yin) energy which keeps the (Yang) machine of the body running properly.

Massage is a very simple Qigong practice which can increase the Qi and blood circulation in the body. It is widely studied and practiced in Chinese medicine and martial arts. Because massage can regulate and adjust the Qi circulating in the body, it is used not only to maintain health and prevent illness, but also to heal injuries and cure many illnesses.

Chinese massage can be classified into four categories: relaxation massage for health (Pu Tong An Mo), Tui Na (push-grab) massage for treating injury and some illnesses, Dian Xue (cavity press) massage for illnesses, and Qi healing (Wai Qi Liao Fa). We will cover the discussion of these categories in two volumes. In the first volume, we will review the basic theory of Qigong and survey the history of massage in China. In addition, we will introduce the theory and the techniques of general massage and also some techniques for self-massage. In the second volume, we will discuss the other three types of massage separately.

If you are not familiar with the theory and philosophy of Chinese Qigong, we recommend you read the YMAA book "The Root of Chinese Chi Kung" first. It will give you a clear understanding of general Qigong practices.

These two volumes are written for your reference, and are not meant to be the authority on massage. Do not hesitate to compare them with what you have learned from other sources about Chinese and other types of massage.

My knowledge of techniques and theory, which is primarily in the fields of relaxation massage, Tui Na, and some Dian Xue, comes from my White Crane martial arts master. My knowledge of the deeper aspects of Dian Xue massage, which is used for curing illness, is limited. Most of the information on this subject in this book was compiled from several Chinese publications. I hope that those who are more proficient in this field will come forth and share their understanding and experience.

Finally, in order to be consistent with international usage, we have started using the Pinyin system for spelling Chinese words. We hope that this will be more convenient for those readers who consult other Chinese books. However, in order to avoid confusion, commonly accepted spellings of names will not be changed, such as Tamkang College and Taipei. In addition, the spelling which individuals have chosen for their names will not be changed either, such as my name, Yang Jwing-Ming, or Wen-Ching Wu, etc.

CONTENTS

PART ONE

INTRODUCTION

Chapter 1
General Concepts

1-1. Introduction

Although health has always been one of mankind's main concerns, most people aren't very interested in learning how to keep themselves healthy. It seems that we don't really appreciate our health until we have lost it. The fact is, the best way to stay healthy is to prevent sickness from occurring. Your body is like a machine in that performing preventive maintenance is cheaper than waiting for something to go wrong and then fixing it. Furthermore, in many cases it is impossible to bring the body back to the state it was in before the sickness. Also, when you are sick your body tends to degenerate faster than it usually does in the normal process of aging.

You may have noticed that many illnesses do not pop up overnight. In fact, many of them are caused by our bad habits and the way we abuse our bodies. Often, unhealthy conditions are made worse by our ignoring what is going on in our own bodies. Too many people think that their health is their physician's concern and responsibility, and not their own. In fact, if you are willing to pay attention to your own state of health you can probably cut your health problems in half.

Since ancient times, Chinese medicine and Qigong have been very much concerned with maintaining health and preventing illness. According to Chinese medicine, the human body has two components: the Qi body (inner energy body, or Yin body) and the physical body (manifestation body, or Yang body). Chinese medicine considers the Qi body to be the foundation of the Yang body, and the root of health and longevity. This means that Yin energy is the origin of life, and it makes the growth of Yang possible. When Yin energy weakens or suddenly increases, the change is manifested in the Yang (physical) body. If the imbalance persists, physical damage or even failure to function will occur in the body.

For example, if you are not feeling well and go to see a Western physician, he will examine you and perhaps take X-rays. If he cannot find any defect or damage in your physical body, he will probably tell you that you are perfectly healthy, or that what you feel is only in your mind. However, when you go to see a traditional Chinese physician, he will first gauge the Qi levels of the twelve primary Qi channels which are related to your internal organs. If the physician finds any abnormality in your Qi circulation, he will use acupuncture, herbs, massage, or other methods to adjust it. This will prevent physical damage from occurring. This concept is very different from that of Western physicians, who wait for visible, physical damage to actually occur before they consider you to be sick.

Another way in which traditional Chinese medicine differs from Western medicine is that Chinese medicine treats the entire body as a whole, rather than only treating that part of the body which is sick. For example, if there is a problem with the liver, the Western physician will treat it as a liver problem only. However, in Chinese medicine the treatment will be very different, for the physician will be concerned with how the problem in the liver arose. What is the root of the abnormal Qi circulation in the liver? Is it because the kidney Qi is too Yang, or is it because the heart Qi is too Yin? If you want to understand the roots of a problem with an organ, you need to know how it relates to all the other organs. According to Chinese medicine, all of the internal organs are related and connected through the Qi, and they affect each other's functioning. Therefore, in order to treat a problem, the physician must find the source of the sickness, and not just treat the symptoms. If the cause of the illness is not removed, the illness can return.

For these reasons, Chinese medicine and Qigong are greatly concerned with maintaining the Yin/Yang balance in the organs and maintaining and improving the Qi circulation in the body. For thousands of years, Qigong massage has proven to be one of the safest and most efficient ways of doing this, and thereby maintaining health and preventing sickness.

Massage is a natural human instinct. When you have pain in some part of your body, your first, natural reaction is to rub it with your hand to reduce the pain. In the beginning, people probably didn't pay much attention to how the pain was released. They simply recognized that massage could reduce pain, relax the patient, increase energy and vitality, and even cure many kinds of sickness.

No one country can claim to have invented the art of massage. Almost every culture in the world has developed or adopted massage techniques at some point in its history. Although the techniques may be somewhat different, and the depth of the theory varies widely, the major purpose of massage treatment - to increase circulation of fluids and energy in the body and improve health - is the same.

The Chinese people have been practicing and researching massage for more than four thousand years, and have developed a comprehensive and consistent theory of massage treatment which is closely integrated with the larger fields of Chinese medicine and Qigong theory. They have tried to answer such questions as: In what ways can massage benefit people? How is Qi (internal energy) related to massage? What is the best treatment in specific cases?

Over the years, many different schools of massage have sprung up, and countless techniques have been developed based on their experience in treatments. However, the differences in the techniques of each school do not matter, since the theory and approach remain the same. Therefore, it is extremely important for you to understand the **WHY**, **WHAT**, and **HOW**. If you simply learn the techniques of massage without knowing the root theory and principles, your knowledge will be restricted to the branches and flowers, and your development will be limited.

To understand Chinese massage, the first question you must ask is: How does Chinese massage differ from Western massage? Chinese massage is commonly called Qigong massage, because it is based on affecting the energetic (Qi) system, as well as the circulatory systems of blood and lymph. (Remember Chinese medicine holds that imbalances or blockages in the Qi circulation system are the root of the body's illnesses.) Therefore, in order to effectively use massage to help the patient recover from sickness, the physician must study Qi, understand the Qi circulatory system in the body, train their own Qi, and learn how to use their Qi while massaging in order to help the patient to regain Qi balance. Massage is classified as one of the major fields of Qigong in China, and requires a long period of concentrated study. You can see that Chinese Qigong massage was developed for healing, rather than just relaxation and enjoyment. If you wish to start learning basic Qigong theory, you can start with the YMAA book "The Root of Chinese Chi Kung."

The second question you need to ask is: How does Chinese massage differ from Japanese Shiatsu massage? If you investigate the Japanese culture, you will find that much of it originated in China. This is especially true with regard to medicine and religion. The study of Qi and Chinese medical practices such as acupuncture have been major influences on Japanese culture, and Shiatsu is one of the results of this. Once you have read this book you will realize that Japanese Shiatsu massage is actually part of Chinese cavity press or acupressure massage, which is discussed in the second volume of this book. Naturally, because of several hundred years of separate development, many techniques and theories of treatment are somewhat different. It may therefore be worthwhile to compare the two arts, so that you can choose the best techniques for your practice.

Qigong massage has proven to be effective in treating injuries and illnesses, although, in many cases, it does not get results as fast as Western medicine. However, it does have a number of advantages: 1. There are no side effects; 2. It can correct problems at their root and in a natural way; 3. Unlike Western medicine, it does not use chemicals, which all too often prove to be addictive and enslaving; and 4. Massage increases your awareness and understanding of your bodies (both the physical and the energy bodies). Knowing yourself better is the key to preventing illness.

Please remember, however, that Western medicine has many strong points, and you should take advantage of them. The wisest way is to coordinate the oriental and the Western ways. Of course, to do this you need to have some knowledge of both approaches.

At this point in human history we have the greatest opportunity so far to communicate with each other freely and openly. If we continue to adhere only to the knowledge which our own culture has developed, and ignore all that has been developed in different cultures, then our minds are sure to be stuck in the ancient past.

Next we will review the concepts of Qi and Qigong. In the third section we will summarize the different categories of Chinese Qigong massage. In the fourth section we will survey the history of Chinese Qigong massage, and in the last section we will discuss how to use this book.

1-2. Qi, Qigong, and Man

Before we discuss the relationship of Qi to the human body, we should first define Qi and Qigong. We will first discuss the general concept of Qi, including both the traditional understanding and the modern scientific viewpoint, and then we will use the modern concepts to explain Qigong. If you would like to investigate these subjects in more detail, please refer to the YMAA book "The Root of Chinese Chi Kung."

A General Definition of Qi

Qi is the energy or natural force which fills the universe. The Chinese have traditionally believed that there are three major powers in the universe. These Three Powers (San Cai) are Heaven (Tian), Earth (Di), and Man (Ren). Heaven (the sky or universe) has Heaven Qi (Tian Qi), the most important of the three, which is made up of the forces which the heavenly bodies exert on the earth, such as sunshine, moonlight, the moon's gravity, and the energy from the stars. In ancient times, the Chinese believed that weather, climate, and natural disasters were governed by Heaven Qi. Chinese people still refer to the weather as Tian Qi (Heaven Qi). Every energy field strives to stay in balance, so whenever the Heaven Qi loses its balance, it tries to rebalance itself. Then the wind must blow, rain must fall, even tornados or hurricanes must happen in order for the Heaven Qi to reach a new energy balance.

Under Heaven Qi, is Earth Qi. It is influenced and controlled by Heaven Qi. For example, too much rain will force a river to flood or change its path. Without rain, the plants will die. The Chinese believe that Earth Qi is made up of lines and patterns of energy, as well as the earth's magnetic field and the heat concealed underground. These energies must also balance, otherwise disasters such as earthquakes will occur. When the Qi of the earth is balanced, plants will grow and animals thrive.

Finally, within the Earth Qi, each individual person, animal, and plant has its own Qi field, which always seeks to be balanced. When any individual thing loses its Qi balance, it will sicken, die, and decompose. All natural things, including mankind and our Human Qi, grow within and are influenced by the natural cycles of Heaven Qi and Earth Qi. Throughout the history of Qigong, people have been most interested in Human Qi and its relationship with Heaven Qi and Earth Qi.

In China, Qi is defined as any type of energy which is able to demonstrate power and strength. This energy can be electricity, magnetism, heat, or light. In China, electric power is called "Dian Qi" (electric Qi), and heat is called "Re Qi" (heat Qi). When a person is alive, his body's energy is called "Ren Qi" (human Qi).

Qi is also commonly used to express the energy state of something, especially living things. As mentioned before, the weather is called "Tian Qi" (heaven Qi) because it indicates the energy state of the heavens. When a thing is alive it has "Huo Qi" (vital Qi), and when it is dead it has "Si Qi" (dead Qi) or "Gui Qi" (ghost Qi). When a person is righteous and has the spiritual strength to do good, he is said to have "Zheng Qi" (Normal Qi or Righteous Qi). The spiritual state or morale of an army is called "Qi Shi" (energy state).

You can see that the word Qi has a wider and more general definition than most people think. It does not refer only to the energy circulating in the human body. Furthermore, the word "Qi" can represent the energy itself, and it can also be used to express the manner or state of the energy. It is important to understand this when you practice Qigong, so that your mind is not channeled into a narrow understanding of Qi, which would limit your future understanding and development.

A Narrow Definition of Qi

Now that you understand the general definition of Qi, let us look at how Qi is defined in Qigong society today. As mentioned before, among the Three Powers, the Chinese have been most concerned with the Qi which is related to our health and longevity. Therefore, after four thousand years of emphasizing Human Qi, when people mention Qi they usually mean the Qi circulating in our bodies.

If we look at the Chinese medical and Qigong documents that were written about two thousand years ago, the word "Qi" was written "炁." This character is constructed of two words, "旡" on the top, which means "nothing;" and " 灬 " on the bottom, which means "fire." This means that the word Qi was actually written as "no fire" in ancient times. If we go back through Chinese medical and Qigong history, it is not hard to understand this expression.

In ancient times, what the Chinese physicians or Qigong practitioners were looking for in their practice was actually the Yin-Yang balance of the Qi which was circulating in the body. When this goal was reached, there was "no fire" in the internal organs. This concept is very simple. According to Chinese medicine, each of our internal organs needs to receive a specific amount of Qi to function properly. If an organ receives an improper amount of Qi (usually too much, i.e., too Yang), it will start to malfunction, and, in time, physical damage will occur. Therefore, the goal of the medical or Qigong practitioner was to attain a state of "no fire," which eventually became the word Qi.

However, in more recent publications, the Qi of "no fire" has been replaced by the word " 氣," which is again constructed of two words, " 气" which means "air," and " 米" which means "rice." This shows that later practitioners realized that the Qi circulating in our bodies is produced mainly by the inhalation of air and the consumption of food (rice). (Air is called Kong Qi, which means literally "space energy".)

For a long time, people were confused about just what type of energy was circulating in our bodies. Many people believed that it was heat, others considered it to be electricity, and many others assumed that it was a mixture of heat, electricity, and light.

This confusion lasted until about fifteen years ago, when the concept of Qi gradually became clear. If we think carefully about what we know from science, we can see that (except possibly for gravity) there is actually only one type of energy in this universe, and that is electromagnetic energy. This means that light (electromagnetic waves) and heat (infrared waves) are also part of electromagnetic energy. This makes it very clear that the Qi circulating in our bodies is actually "bioelectricity," and that our body is a "living electromagnetic field."(*1) This field is affected by our thoughts, feelings, activities, the food we eat, the quality of the air we breathe, our lifestyle, the natural energy that surrounds us, and also the unnatural energy which modern science inflicts upon us.

Next, let us define Qigong. Once you understand what Qigong is, you will be able to better understand the role that Qigong massage plays in Chinese medicine and Qigong society.

A General Definition of Qigong

We have explained that Qi is energy, and that it is found in the heavens, in the earth, and in every living thing. In China, the word "Gong" is often used instead of "Gongfu" (or Kung Fu), which means energy and time. Any study or training which requires a lot of energy and time to learn or to accomplish is called Gongfu. The term can be applied to any special skill or study as long as it requires time, energy, and patience. Therefore, **THE CORRECT DEFINITION OF QIGONG IS ANY TRAINING OR STUDY DEALING WITH QI WHICH TAKES A LONG TIME AND A LOT OF EFFORT**. You can see from this definition that Qigong is a science which studies the energy in nature. The main difference between this energy science and Western energy science is that Qigong focuses on the inner energy of human beings, while Western energy science pays more attention to the energy outside of the human body. When you study Qigong, it is worthwhile to also consider the modern, scientific point of view, and not restrict yourself to only the traditional beliefs.

The Chinese have studied Qi for thousands of years. Some of the information on the patterns and cycles of nature has been recorded in books, one of which is the "Yi Jing" (Book of Changes; 1122 B.C.). When the "Yi Jing" was written, the Chinese people, as mentioned earlier, believed that natural power included Tian (Heaven), Di (Earth), and Ren (Man). These are called "San Cai" (The Three Powers) and are manifested by the three Qi's: Heaven Qi, Earth Qi, and Human Qi. These three facets of nature have their definite rules and cycles. The rules never change, and the cycles repeat regularly. The Chinese people used an understanding of these natural principles and the "Yi Jing" to calculate the changes of natural Qi. This calculation is called "Bagua" (The Eight Trigrams). From the Eight Trigrams are derived the 64 hexagrams. Therefore, the "Yi Jing" was probably the first book which taught the Chinese people about Qi and its variations in nature and man. The relationship of the Three Natural Powers and their Qi variations were later discussed extensively in the book "Qi Hua Lun" (Theory of Qi's Variation).

Understanding Heaven Qi is very difficult, and it was especially so in ancient times when the science was just developing. But since nature is always repeating itself, the experiences accumulated over the years have made it possible to trace the natural patterns. Understanding the rules and cycles of "Tian Shi" (heavenly timing) will help you to understand natural changes of the seasons, climate, weather, rain, snow, drought, and all other natural occurrences. If you observe carefully, you will be able to see many of these routine patterns and cycles caused by the rebalancing of the Qi fields. Among the natural cycles are those which repeat every day, month, or year, as well as cycles of twelve years and sixty years.

Earth Qi is a part of Heaven Qi. If you can understand the rules and the structure of the earth, you will be able to understand how mountains and rivers are formed, how plants grow, how rivers move, what part of the country is best for someone, where to build a house and which direction it should face so that it is a healthy place to live, and many other things related to the earth. In China today there are people, called "Di Li Shi" (geomancy teachers) or "Feng Shui Shi" (wind water teachers), who make their living this way. The term Feng Shui is commonly used because the location and character of the wind and water in a landscape are the most important factors in evaluating a location. These experts use the accumulated body of geomantic knowledge and the "Yi Jing" to help people make important decisions such as where and how to build a house, where to bury their dead, and how to rearrange or redecorate homes and offices so that they are better places to live and work in. Many people even believe that setting up a store or business according to the guidance of Feng Shui can make it more prosperous.

Among the three Qi's, Human Qi is probably the one studied most thoroughly. The study of Human Qi covers a large number of different subjects. The Chinese people believe that Human Qi is affected and controlled by Heaven Qi and Earth Qi, and that they in fact determine your destiny. Therefore, if you understand the relationship between nature and people, in addition to understanding human relations (Ren Shi), you will be able to predict wars, the destiny of a country, a person's desires and temperament, and even their future. The people who practice this profession are called "Suan Ming Shi" (calculate life teachers).

However, the greatest achievement in the study of Human Qi is in regard to health and longevity. Since Qi is the source of life, if you understand how Qi functions and know how to regulate it correctly, you should be able to live a long and healthy life. Remember that you are part of nature, and you are channeled into the cycles of nature. If you go against this natural cycle, you may become sick, so it is in your best interest to follow the way of nature. This is the meaning of "Dao," which can be translated as "The Natural Way."

Many different aspects of Human Qi have been researched, including acupuncture, acupressure, herbal treatment, meditation, and Qigong exercises. The use of acupuncture, acupressure, and herbal treatment to adjust Human Qi flow has become the root of Chinese medical science. Meditation and moving Qigong exercises are used widely by the Chinese people to improve their health or even to cure certain illnesses. In addition, Daoists and Buddhists use meditation and Qigong exercises in their pursuit of enlightenment.

In conclusion, the study of any of the aspects of Qi including Heaven Qi, Earth Qi, and Human Qi should be called Qigong. However, since the term is usually used today only in reference to the cultivation of Human Qi through meditation and exercises, we will only use it in this narrower sense to avoid confusion.

A Narrow Definition of Qigong

As mentioned earlier, the narrow definition of Qi is "the energy circulating in the human body." Therefore, the narrow definition of Qigong is "the study of the Qi circulating in the human body." Because our bodies are part of nature, the narrow definition of Qigong should also include the study of how our bodies relate to Heaven Qi and Earth Qi. Chinese Qigong consists today of several different fields: acupuncture, herbs for regulating human Qi, martial arts Qigong, Qigong massage, Qigong exercises, Qigong healing, and religious enlightenment Qigong. Naturally, these fields are mutually related, and in many cases cannot be separated.

The Chinese have discovered that the human body has twelve major channels and eight vessels through which the Qi circulates. The twelve channels are like rivers which distribute Qi throughout the body, and also connect the extremities (fingers and toes) to the internal organs. Here you should understand that the "internal organs" of Chinese medicine do not necessarily correspond to the physical organs as understood in the West, but rather to a set of clinical functions similar to each other, and related to the organ system. The eight vessels, which are often referred to as the extraordinary vessels, function like reservoirs and regulate the distribution and circulation of Qi in your body.

When the Qi in the eight reservoirs is full and strong, the Qi in the rivers is strong and will be regulated efficiently. When there is stagnation in any of these twelve channels or rivers, the Qi which flows to the body's extremities and to the internal organs will be abnormal, and illness may develop. You should understand that every channel has its particular Qi flow strength, and every channel is different. All of these different levels of Qi strength are affected by your mind, the weather, the time of day, the food you have eaten, and even your mood. For example, when the weather is dry the Qi in the lungs will tend to be more positive than when it is moist. When you are angry, the Qi flow in your liver channel will be abnormal. The Qi strength in the different channels varies throughout the day in a regular cycle, and at any particular time one channel is strongest. For example, between 11 AM and 1 PM the Qi flow in the heart channel is the strongest. Furthermore, the Qi level of the same organ can be different from one person to another.

Whenever the Qi flow in the twelve rivers or channels is not normal, the eight reservoirs will regulate the Qi flow and bring it back to normal. For example, when you experience a sudden shock, the Qi flow in the bladder immediately becomes deficient. Normally, the reservoir will immediately regulate the Qi in this channel so that you recover from the shock. However, if the reservoir Qi is also deficient, or if the effect of the shock is too great and there is not enough time to regulate the Qi, the bladder will suddenly contract, causing unavoidable urination.

When a person is sick because of an injury, his Qi level tends to be either too positive (excessive, Yang) or too negative (deficient, Yin). A Chinese physician would either use a prescription of herbs to adjust the Qi, or else he would insert acupuncture needles at various spots on the channels to inhibit the flow in some channels and stimulate the flow in others, so that balance can be restored. However, there is another alternative, and that is to use certain physical and mental exercises to adjust the Qi. In other words, to use Qigong.

The above discussion is only to offer an idea of the narrow definition of Qigong. In fact, when people talk about Qigong today, most of the time they are referring to the mental and physical exercises that work with the Qi.

A Modern Definition of Qi

It is important that you know about the progress that has been made by modern science in the study of Qi. This will keep you from getting stuck in the ancient concepts and level of understanding.

In ancient China, people had very little knowledge of electricity. They only knew from acupuncture that when a needle was inserted into the acupuncture cavities, some kind of energy other than heat was produced which often caused a shock or a tickling sensation. It was not until the last few decades, when the Chinese people were more acquainted with electromagnetic science, that they began to recognize that this energy circulating in the body, which they called Qi, might be the same thing as what today's science calls "bioelectricity."

It is understood now that the human body is constructed of many different electrically conductive materials, and that it forms a living electromagnetic field and circuit. Electromagnetic energy is continuously being generated in the human body through the biochemical reaction of food and air, and circulated by the electromagnetic forces (EMF) generated within the body.

In addition, you are also constantly being affected by external electromagnetic fields such as that of the earth, or the electrical fields generated by clouds. When you practice Chinese medicine or Qigong, you need to be aware of these outside factors and take them into account.

Countless experiments have been conducted in China, Japan, and other countries to study how external magnetic or electrical fields can affect and adjust the body's Qi field. Many acupuncturists use magnets and electricity in their treatments. They attach a magnet to the skin over a cavity and leave it there for a period of time. The magnetic field gradually affects the Qi circulation in that channel. Alternatively, they insert needles into cavities and then run an electric current through the needle to reach the Qi channels directly. Although many experimenters have claimed a degree of success in their experiments, none has been able to publish any detailed and convincing proof of the results, or give a good explanation of the theory behind the experiment. As with many other attempts to explain the How and Why of acupuncture, conclusive proof is elusive, and many unanswered questions remain. Of course, this theory is quite new, and it will probably take a lot more study and research before it is verified and completely understood. At present, there are many conservative acupuncturists who are skeptical.

To untie this knot, we must look at what modern Western science has discovered about bioelectromagnetic energy. Many bioelectricity-related reports have been published, and frequently the results are closely related to what is experienced in Chinese Qigong training and medical science. For example, during the electrophysiological research of the 1960's, several investigators discovered that bones are piezoelectric; that is, when they are stressed, mechanical energy is converted to electrical energy in the form of electric current.(*1) This might explain one of the practices of Marrow Washing Qigong in which the stress on the bones and muscles is increased in certain ways to increase the Qi circulation.

Dr. Robert O. Becker has done important work in this field. His book "The Body Electric"(*2) reports on much of the research concerning the body's electric field. It is presently believed that food and air are the fuels which generate the electricity in the body through biochemical reaction. This electricity, which is circulated throughout the entire body through electrically conductive tissue, is one of the main energy sources which keep the cells of the physical body alive.

Whenever you have an injury or are sick, your body's electrical circulation is affected. If this circulation of electricity stops, you die. But bioelectric energy not only maintains life, it is also responsible for repairing physical damage. Many researchers have sought ways of using external electrical or magnetic fields to speed up the body's recovery from physical injury. Richard Leviton reports that: "Researchers at Loma Linda University's School of Medicine in California have found, following studies in sixteen countries with over 1,000 patients, that low-frequency, low-intensity magnetic energy has been successful in treating chronic pain related to tissue ischemia, and also worked in clearing up slow-healing ulcers, and in 90 percent of patients tested, raised blood flow significantly."(*3)

Mr. Leviton also reports that every cell of the body functions like an electric battery and is able to store electric charges. He reports that: "Other biomagnetic investigators take an even closer look to find out what is happening, right down to the level of the blood, the organs, and the individual cell, which they regard as "a small electric battery"."(*3) This has convinced me that our entire body is just like a big battery which is assembled from millions of small batteries. All of these batteries together form the human electromagnetic field.

Furthermore, much of the research on the body's electrical field relates to acupuncture. For example, Dr. Becker reports that the conductivity of the skin is much higher at acupuncture cavities, and that it is now possible to locate them precisely by measuring the skin's conductivity. Many of these reports prove that the acupuncture which has been done in China for thousands of years is reasonable and scientific.

Some researchers use the theory of the body's electricity to explain many of the ancient "miracles" which have been attributed to the practice of Qigong. A report by Albert L. Huebner states: "These demonstrations of body electricity in human beings may also offer a new explanation of an ancient healing practice. If weak external fields can produce powerful physiological effects, it may be that fields from human tissues in one person are capable of producing clinical improvements in another. In short, the method of healing known as the laying on of hands could be an especially subtle form of electrical stimulation."(*1)

Another frequently reported phenomenon is that when a Qigong practitioner has reached a high level of development, a halo would appear behind and/or around their head during meditation. This is commonly seen in paintings of Jesus Christ, the Buddha, and various Oriental gods. Frequently the light is pictured as surrounding the whole body. This phenomenon may again be explained by the body electric theory. When a person has cultivated their Qi (electricity) to a high level, the Qi may be led to accumulate in the head. This Qi may then interact with the oxygen molecules in the air, and ionize them, causing them to glow.

Although the link between the theory of the body electric and the Chinese theory of Qi is becoming more accepted and better proven, there are still many questions to be answered. For example, how can the mind lead Qi (electricity)? How actually does the mind generate an EMF (electromagnetic force) to circulate the electricity in the body? How is the human electromagnetic field affected by the multitude of other electric fields which surround us, such as radio and television waves, or the fields generated by household electrical wiring or electrical appliances? How can we readjust our electromagnetic fields and survive in outer space or on other planets where the magnetic field is completely different from the earth's? You can see that the future of Qigong and bioelectric science is a challenging and exciting one. It is about time that we started to use modern technology to understand the inner energy world which has been for the most part ignored by Western society.

A Modern Definition of Qigong

If you now accept that the inner energy (Qi) circulating in our bodies is bioelectricity, then we can easily create a definition of Qigong based on the concept of electricity.

Let us assume that the circuit shown in Figure 1-1 is similar to the circuit in our bodies. Unfortunately, although we now have a certain degree of understanding of this circuit from acupuncture, we still do not know in detail exactly what the body's circuit looks like. We know that there are twelve primary Qi channels (Qi rivers) and eight vessels (Qi reservoirs) in our body. There are also thousands of small Qi channels which allow the Qi to reach the skin and the bone marrow. In this circuit, the twelve internal organs are connected and mutually related through these channels.

If you look at the electric circuit in the illustration, you will see that:

1. The Qi channels are like the wires which carry the electric current.
2. The internal organs are like the electrical components such as resistors and solenoids.

Figure 1-1. The human bioelectric circuit is similar to an electric circuit.

3.   The Qi vessels are like a capacitor, which regulates the current in the circuit.

How do you keep this electrical circuit functioning most efficiently? Your first concern is with the resistance of the wire which carries the current. In a machine, you want to use a wire which has a high level of conductivity and low resistance, otherwise the current may melt the wire. Therefore, the wire should be of a material like copper or perhaps even gold. In your body, you want to keep the current flowing smoothly. This means that your first task is to remove anything which interferes with the flow and cause stagnation. Fat has low conductivity, so you should use diet and exercise to remove excess fat from your body. You should also learn how to relax your physical body, because this opens all of the Qi channels. This is why relaxation is the first goal in Taijiquan and many Qigong exercises.

Your next concern in maintaining a healthy electrical circuit is the components - your internal organs. If you do not have the correct level of current in your organs, they will either burn out from too much current (Yang) or malfunction because of a deficient level of current (Yin). In order to avoid these problems in a machine, you use a capacitor to regulate the current. Whenever there is too much current, the capacitor absorbs and stores the excess, and whenever the current is weak, the capacitor supplies current to raise the level. The eight Qi vessels are your body's capacitor. Qigong is concerned with learning how to increase the level of Qi in these vessels so that they will be able to supply current when needed and keep the internal organs functioning smoothly. This is especially important as you get older and your Qi level is generally lower.

Finally, in order to have a healthy circuit, you have to be concerned with the components themselves. If any of them are not strong and of good quality, the entire circuit will have problems. This means that the final concern in Qigong practice is how to maintain or even rebuild the health of your internal organs. Before we go any further, we should point out that there is an important difference between the circuit shown in the diagram and the Qi circuit in our bodies. This difference is that the human body is alive, and, with the proper Qi nourishment, all of the cells can be regrown and the state of health improved. For example, if you are able to jog about three miles today, and if you keep jogging regularly and gradually increase the distance, eventually you will be able to easily jog five miles. This is because your body rebuilds and readjusts itself to fit the circumstances.

This means that, if we are able to increase the Qi flow through our internal organs, they can become stronger and healthier. Naturally, the increase in Qi must be slow and gradual so that the organs can readjust to it. In order to increase the Qi flow in your body, you need to work with the EMF (electromagnetic force) in your body. If you do not know what EMF is, please imagine two containers filled with water and connected by a tube. If both containers have the same water level, then the water will not flow. However, if one side is higher than the other, the water will flow from that container to the other. In electricity, this potential difference is called electromagnetic force. Naturally, the higher the EMF is, the stronger the current will flow.

You can see from this discussion that the key to effective Qigong practice is, in addition to removing resistance from the Qi channels, learning how to increase the EMF in your body. Now let us see what the sources of EMF in the body are, so that we may use them to increase the flow of bioelectricity. Generally speaking, there are five major sources:

1. **Natural Energy.** Since your body is constructed of electrically conductive material, its electromagnetic field is always affected by the sun, the moon, clouds, the earth's magnetic field, and by the other energies around you. The major influences are the sun's radiation, the moon's gravity, and the earth's magnetic field. These affect your Qi circulation significantly, and are responsible for the pattern of your Qi circulation since you were formed. We are now also being greatly affected by the energy generated by modern technology, such as the electromagnetic waves generated by radio, TV, microwave ovens, computers, and many other things.

2. **Food and Air.** In order to maintain life, we take in food and air essence through our mouth and nose. These essences are then

converted into Qi through biochemical reaction in the chest and digestive system (called the Triple Burner in Chinese medicine). When Qi is converted from the essence, an EMF is generated which circulates the Qi throughout the body. Consequently a major part of Qigong is devoted to getting the proper kinds of food and fresh air.

3. Thinking. The human mind is the most important and efficient source of bioelectric EMF. Any time you move to do something you must first generate an idea (Yi). This idea generates the EMF and leads the Qi to energize the appropriate muscles to carry out the desired motion. The more you can concentrate, the stronger the EMF you can generate, and the stronger the flow of Qi you can lead. Naturally, the stronger the flow of Qi you lead to the muscles, the more they will be energized. Because of this, the mind is considered the most important factor in Qigong training.

4. Exercise. Exercise converts the food essence (fat) stored in your body into Qi, and therefore builds up the EMF. Many Qigong styles have been created which utilize movement for this purpose.

5. Converting Pre-birth Essence into Qi. The hormones produced by our endocrine glands are referred to as "Pre-birth essence" in Chinese medicine. They can be converted into Qi to stimulate the functioning of our physical body, thereby increasing our vitality. Balancing horone production when you are young and increasing its production when you are old are important subjects in Chinese Qigong.

In this section we have attempted to explain the general concepts behind Qi and Qigong. The same principles also apply to Qigong massage, whose goal is also to maintain and improve Qi circulation so that you can stay healthy, heal injuries, and fight illness. Since Qigong massage is only a branch of Chinese Qigong, it would be very helpful for you to also study other types of Qigong which have grown from the same root; you would then have a better overview of the whole field of Qigong.

1-3. Definition and Categories of Qigong Massage

Because there are so many categories of Chinese Qigong massage, and it is very easy to become confused, we will first define each one of them and explain its scope, boundaries, and purposes.

Chinese massage is commonly called "An Mo." "An" means "press" and "Mo" means "rub." Chinese massage is constructed around the two major techniques **PRESS** and **RUB**, though, of course, many other techniques are also used. Chinese massage can be broken down into four major categories, depending upon the specialized techniques which it uses for its particular purposes. They are Pu Tong An Mo (General Massage), Tui Na An Mo (Push Grab Massage), Dian Xue An Mo (Cavity Press Massage), and Qi An Mo (Qi Massage).

In this section, we will define each category, briefly review its basic theory, and point out how it differs from the other categories. However, I would like to point out here that, because the basic theories and principles are the same for all the categories, many masseurs are familiar with more than one category.

1. Pu Tong An Mo (General Massage):

The most common and popular category of massage in China is called "Pu Tong An Mo" (General Massage). In the West it is sometimes translated as "Relaxation Massage." The goals of general or relaxation massage are probably the simplest, as are the techniques. Because this kind of massage does not deal with injuries or illness, no in-depth knowledge of the Qi channels and Chinese medical theory is required. This category is also the safest.

In all of the larger cities throughout the Orient are many masseurs whom people patronize to relax and recover from fatigue. Many of these masseurs are blind. There are several reasons for this: 1. Blind people have a more acute sense of touch, and can usually massage better than sighted people. 2. Since blind people cannot see your body, there was less shame in being massaged by them in the older, puritanical societies. 3. Massage was the easiest way for a blind person to earn a living. In Oriental cities, it used to be very common to hear the sound of a flute in the evening. That was how blind masseurs advertised that they were looking for customers. These people usually were not skilled in Tui Na or Dian Xue. They simply massaged the muscles to help the customer relax. This "Muscle Grabbing Massage" is called "Zhua Long," which means "Grabbing the Dragon." "Dragon" here refers to the muscles or tendons.

The purposes of this kind of massage are:

A. Relaxation. This includes both physical and mental relaxation. Even if you aren't involved in strenuous physical activity, worry, stress, and responsibility can cause mental tension. Physical tension can be caused by incorrect posture, worry, or even intense thinking. Tension causes your Qi and blood circulation to become stagnant. When this condition persists it can lead to insomnia, nervous breakdown, and even physical damage because of insufficient Qi and blood nourishment. Relaxation or general massage can calm your agitated mind, relax your physical body, and allow the Qi and blood to circulate smoothly.

B. Recovery from Fatigue. Recovery from fatigue refers primarily to physical fatigue from hard labor or exercise. Acid accumulates in the muscles, and causes aches and muscular soreness. General massage is very effective in improving Qi and blood circulation, which helps to remove the accumulated acid.

C. Preventing Illness. One of the main purposes of relaxation massage is the prevention of illness by smoothing out the Qi and blood circulation before any physical damage can occur. Smooth Qi and blood circulation is essential to maintaining the normal functioning of our thinking and our physical body. This is the primary difference between relaxaton massage and the other three categories of massage, which are used to treat injuries and illness.

D. Slowing Down Aging. Maintaining smooth Qi and blood circulation is the key to slowing down the aging process. As we grow older, our Qi and blood circulation slows down and becomes more stagnant. General massage helps to overcome this.

E. Speeding Recovery from Sudden Environmental Qi Disturbances. When our environment changes suddenly, the Qi in our bodies will often not be able to change as quickly. For example, when the weather changes suddenly, our bodies cannot adjust quickly enough, and we may get sick. This problem is especially serious today when modern transportation can bring you from one part of the world to another in a very short time. The sudden changes in the time of day, weather, and altitude can cause problems such as jet lag. General or relaxation massage helps the body to adjust itself to these changes.

F. Enjoyment. The last purpose of relaxation or general massage is enjoyment. Many people get massaged even when they do not have any unhealthy symptoms. Their reason is very simple: massage makes you feel good. This feeling comes mostly from the mind and the relaxation of the physical body. However, there is another reason, and that is the emotional comfort which one obtains from massage. Many people massage each other looking for the emotional balance that comes from touching and being touched by another human being. Most of the time the people involved know each other. This is similar to why we hug lovers and friends.

2. Tui Na An Mo (Push Grab Massage):
"Tui Na An Mo" is also often simply called "Tui Na." The two words mean "push" and "grab to control," and refer to the two main techniques. Tui Na has two main purposes. The first is for treating injuries, and the second is for treating illnesses, especially of small children. People are often confused about the differences between general massage and Tui Na massage, especially since most practitioners of Tui Na massage are also experts in general massage. However, if you look at the differences in the purposes of these two arts, they are quite easy to distinguish.

The first type of Tui Na is widely practiced by Chinese martial artists because they emphasize techniques for treating injuries which commonly occur during training. This kind of Tui Na is often called "Die Da," which means "Fall Strike," to reflect the fact that it specializes in treating injuries caused by falling and being struck. This art treats primarily external injuries such as bruises, ligament damage, Qi stagnation due to old injuries, broken bones, joint dislocations, and so on.

Traditional physicians were also trained in the treatment of injuries. For example, during the Song dynasty (960-1126 A.D.) part of the training of a physician involved bone realignment, and was called "Zheng Gu Ke," or "Align the Bone Category," and in the Ming dynasty (1368-1644 A.D.) the training was called "Jie Gu Ke," which means "Connect Bone Category." You might assume from the names that Zheng Gu and Jie Gu dealt with bone problems exclusively, but this is not the case. Since bone problems are among the most serious external injuries, these two terms were often used to represent Tui Na. This is simply because the physician who knows how to correct bone injuries usually is an expert in all other external injuries. In southern China, Taiwan and Fujian province, Tui Na or Zheng Gu is also commonly called "Cao Jie," which means "Manipulate to Connect." This gives some indication of how difficult it is to determine precisely what a name refers to, and also to the overlap in coverage among the various types of massage.

Ancient documents tell us that Tui Na has been used since the Ming dynasty (1368 A.D.) to cure some illnesses of small children and occasionally adults. The reason for this is very simple. Treatment by acupuncture requires the willing cooperation of the patient as the physician inserts needles, and the patient needs to remain still for a while. This is almost impossible with small children. It is much easier for the physician to use Tui Na techniques to stimulate or sedate the Qi and achieve the same goal as acupuncture. Naturally, the Tui Na masseur must know how to diagnose diseases and evaluate the Qi of the patient, so this type of Tui Na is done mostly by physicians. This does not mean that masters of martial Tui Na do not know how to cure illnesses with Tui Na. In fact, many martial artists were knowledgeable physicians.

3. Dian Xue An Mo (Cavity Press Massage):

The next category of Chinese massage is "Dian Xue An Mo" or simply "Dian Xue," which means literally "point cavity." Dian Xue is commonly translated "acupressure" in the West. This category uses mainly Press and Rub techniques on cavities and certain non-cavity points. According to Chinese medicine, there are more than seven hundred cavities which can be used for acupuncture treatment. Needles are inserted into these cavities to access the channels and adjust the Qi circulation. It was discovered that there are about 108 cavities where finger pressure can access Qi channels. That was the beginning of acupressure. It was also learned that stimulating one of these cavities vigorously would damage the internal organ related to it, a fact which greatly interested the martial artists.

Like acupuncture, cavity press techniques adjust Qi in the channels to make the related organs either more positive or negative. Therefore, Dian Xue An Mo specializes in curing sicknesses caused by Qi imbalance. As you can imagine, physicians contributed greatly to the development of this art. Dian Xue An Mo is the root of Japanese Shiatsu massage.

To use Dian Xue, a physician or a martial artist must have a thorough knowledge of Qi channels and acupuncture, and must be experienced in working directly with Qi. They need to know precisely what treatments are needed for which ailments, and they need to be skilled in applying the correct pressure to the right cavity at the appropriate time of day.

Since both Tui Na and Dian Xue utilize the Qi channels, just what is the difference between them? Tui Na works mainly on the channels while Dian Xue works on the cavities. The pressure used in Dian Xue massage is more penetrating than that used in Tui Na massage, and so, in adults, Dian Xue massage is quicker and more effective. However, Dian Xue is not used much in the treatment of infants, since its potent power can easily injure their internal organs. Also, few physicians possess the required depth of knowledge to effectively use Dian Xue.

According to the available documents, very few martial artists were involved in training Qi before 500 A.D. Since then, however, many have taken it up in order to learn how to disturb an opponent's Qi. The Southern and internal Chinese martial styles are especially known for this. Some of the higher level martial artists also became experts in using the art for healing as well as killing. Because martial artists had to be skilled in Tui Na to cure the external injuries caused by training or combat, high level martial priests or artists were recognized as the real experts in Chinese massage society.

Nowadays, however, acupressure physicians are more popular and easier to find than martial artists who are skilled in healing, and they are usually much more experienced in curing sickness. In addition, many physicians who specialize in Dian Xue massage are also familiar with the Tui Na techniques, and those who use mainly the Tui Na are often experienced in Dian Xue, so the combination term "Dian Xue Tui Na" (Point Cavity Push Grab) is often heard.

4. Qi An Mo (Qi Massage):

The last category of massage is "Qi massage." Qi massage is commonly called "Wai Qi Liao Fa" which means "Curing with External Qi," and is commonly translated "Qigong Healing" in the West today. This term implies that the massage is done through Qi correspondence rather than touch. Because it does not use "press" (An) and "rub" (Mo), it is often not considered to be massage. However, since the goal of Wai Qi Liao Fa is to smooth out the Qi and improve the Qi and blood circulation, which is the same as all other forms of massage, I would like to include it in our discussion.

To understand Qi massage, you must recognize that Qi is the bio-electricity circulating in the body. Because it is electricity, it can be conducted or led through electrical correspondence. Actually, everybody has the ability to do Qi healing. To give an example, when people are sad, their Qi is Yin (deficient). If you hold their hands or hug them, your Qi will nourish them and they will immediately feel better. We have been doing this instinctively for a long time. The only difference between the average person and a Qigong master is that the latter has trained in Qi healing, and can therefore be more effective.

There are two kinds of Qi massage, one which involves touching the skin, and one which does not. Qi massage which uses skin contact is further subdivided into two categories. In the first one, the Qigong master or physician uses Dian Xue massage, but also uses their own Qi to nourish the patient through the cavities if the patient's Qi is too deficient (Yin), or to remove excess Qi through skin contact if there is an excess of Qi (Yang). The practitioner must be sure to get rid of the Qi they have absorbed, or they might be harmed by it. It is therefore important to be highly skilled in Qigong before practicing Qi healing.

The second kind of Qi massage using skin contact is when the practitioner lightly touches the patient's skin and has their Qi correspond with the patient's Qi. This mutual correspondence allows the healer to lead the disordered Qi back into the proper pattern. Again, the practitioner must also know how to keep their own Qi from being unbalanced by the patient's. It is essential in this kind of healing that the healer and the patient cooperate closely with each other.

In the Qi massage which does not use skin contact, the practitioner uses the fingertips or the Laogong cavity in the palm (which is the gate through which one's Qi communicates with the outside world) to focus Qi in a cavity or area of the patient's body. They are able to use their Qi to affect the Qi in the patient, without even touching them. Another method is to move their hands over the patient's body to help them to smooth a disordered pattern of Qi. Theoretically, massage which doesn't use skin contact is safer for the practitioner, since one does not absorb Qi from the patient, which may threaten the health of the practitioner.

You can see that there is some ambiguity as to just what should be included under the term "massage." If your definition of massage depends upon its purpose, then any technique which helps to smooth and improve the Qi and blood circulation should be considered massage. However, if you define massage as using the techniques of Press (An) and Rub (Mo), then there needs to be actual skin contact, and Wai Qi Liao Fa would not be included.

1-4. History of Qigong Massage

Since massage is a natural, instinctive human reaction to pain, injury, and even sickness, we cannot determine when massage really started in any culture. However, every country has its own history of massage. In this section we will only cover the history of massage in China, according to the records and documents which are available today.

When you study the history of massage in China, you need to recognize the various groups which have contributed the most over the past several thousand years. You then need to understand how and why they became involved in massage. Finally, you need to be aware of how much each group has contributed to massage as it is practiced today. With this understanding, you will be able to avoid confusion over the many different categories of massage.

There were four main groups which significantly influenced massage in China: physicians, martial artists, the clergy, and laymen masseurs. Let us first look briefly at each of these groups.

1. Physicians:

When people are injured, they will usually seek out a physician. Massage has always been one of the main methods of treating injuries. It can lessen pain, improve Qi and blood circulation, and release mental tension. All of these can help to effect a rapid recovery. As mentioned earlier, this type of injury treatment is called "Tui Na massage." Later, Tui Na massage eventually developed into a way of treating illnesses in small children.

Acupuncture has also been developing since the beginning of Chinese culture. Out of the principles of acupuncture was developed acupressure or Dian Xue massage (cavity press), which was widely used by physicians. Most of the documents available on this subject were written by physicians. Frequently, massage was discussed together with other methods of treatment such as acupuncture or herbs. The pre-eminence of the physicians was probably attributable to the fact that they were usually the best educated and the most open-minded of the four groups that contributed to the development of massage. In addition, they probably had the most experience. Furthermore, new discoveries and ideas were put into writing, and books spread the new knowledge far and wide. This communication and exchange of techniques brought medical massage to the highest level. In fact, many Chinese physicians were also expert in all categories of Qigong massage.

In the last fifty years, Qi massage, also commonly called Qi healing, has become more popular among physicians in China. It used to be kept secret, and practiced only by Qigong practitioners and physicians who were also expert in Qigong. Since this healing technique has been revealed to the general public, we can confidently predict that it will become more popular and widely accepted during the next fifty years.

2. Martial Artists:

The second largest group of contributors to the development of Chinese massage was the martial artists. Although the history of martial arts massage is not as long as that of medical massage, and there are not as many documents available, it has probably reached a higher level than medical massage in certain areas. This is especially true in the treatment of both internal and external injuries.

How can this have happened? If you look at how and why martial artists developed massage techniques, you will understand why most Chinese people will go to a martial artist to get an injury treated, rather than to a general physician. First, you should understand that martial artists had more experience with injuries than most people, and it was absolutely necessary for them to know how to treat themselves and each other. Tui Na massage was one of the main methods of treatment, and used to be a required course of study for all Chinese martial artists.

Next, you should know that after training long and hard, massage was the best way to get rid of fatigue and eliminate the acid accumulated in the muscles. Massaging each other helped martial artists recover from fatigue, but it also helped them understand the structure of the body and the Qi distribution system. This was very necessary in combat. Therefore, martial artists were often also experts in general and relaxation massage.

The third point which will help you to understand the development of massage in martial society is that massage taught the martial artist precisely where the cavities (vital points) were located. Because most massage points are also used as striking points, massage training was the best way for the student to learn the cavities and experience their depth. When you strike these cavities with power you will cause injury or even death by disturbing the Qi. But you can use the same cavities in healing by applying gentle pressure or rubbing in order to adjust disturbed Qi. Massage was a necessity for any martial artist who wanted to reach the higher levels. Because of this, martial artists who had reached a high level of skill were also experts in cavity press massage for healing. Of course, much of the knowledge of healing could have been obtained from the books available at that time, and many of the martial artists were also physicians. This re-emphasizes the fact that, regardless of how Chinese medicine was developed, it was always based on the same Qi theory, and an understanding of this theory was necessary for reaching the higher levels of the martial arts.

The final point I would like to make is that almost all Chinese martial styles train Qigong. It is necessary for reaching the higher levels of power generation, which is critical for the effective use of techniques in combat. As a result, many martial artists in China become experts in Qigong. One of the best ways to understand Qi and its relationship with the physical body is through massage. Massage helps you to train your Qi, and improves your concentration, which is important for cavity strike techniques.

More than one hundred martial styles have been developed in China over the last five thousand years. Traditionally, each style kept its training theory and fighting techniques secret, and the information was passed down to only a few, trusted students. It was only in the last fifty years that a limited number of books or documents were revealed to the public.

3. Clergy:

The third group that contributed to the development of massage in China was the religious community, mostly Buddhist and Daoist monks. Qigong was part of their training for attaining Buddhahood or enlightenment, and it also included massage. For example, massage is an integral part of the training of Muscle/Tendon Changing (Yi Jin Jing) and Brain/Marrow Washing (Xi Sui Jing). This school of massage was restricted to those within the monastic society. However, some of the massage techniques were revealed to the public in this century by martial artists within the society (e.g., Shaolin and Wudang monks).

4. Laymen:

The last group which contributed to the development of massage is probably the largest, although the level of their practice was the most superficial. The people who gave general, relaxation massages to the general public can be found all over the Orient. They give enjoyable, relaxing massages, and help their clients to release the stress and tension which builds up in daily life. They usually do not pay much attention to using Qi for healing. There are a few books available on this type of massage, but they do not go into the subject of healing very deeply.

Next, we will survey the general history of Chinese massage. Because massage in China is a part of medical treatment and shares the same foundation of Qi theory, it is necessary to understand the development of Chinese medicine when you look at the history of massage. Most of the documents in this section have come from physicians.

In the Xia dynasty (2205-1766 B.C.), when most tools were made of stone,(*4) acupuncturists manipulated their patients' Qi with stone probes (Shi Zhen or Bian Shi) and bone (Gu Zhen), or even thorns. It was recorded in "Shan Hai Jing, Dong Shan Jing" (Mountain Ocean Classic, East Mountain Classic) that: "On the mountain of Gao, there is much jade on the top and many Zhen Shi underneath."(*5) Zhen Shi was later explained by Dr. Shi Guo-Pu: "Zhen Shi is used as a probing needle for curing pain and swelling."(*6) Stone probes (needles), were again explained by Xu Shen in his book "Shuo Wen Jie Zi" (Analysis of Documents with Explanation of Terms) during Han dynasty: "Bian (stone probe), use the stone to pierce the sickness."(*7)

During the Shang dynasty (1766-1122 B.C.), stone tools, including acupuncture needles, were widely replaced by bronze ones. An archeological dig at a late Shang dynasty burial ground called Yin Xu discovered more than 160,000 pieces of turtle shell and animal bone which were covered with written characters. This writing, called "Jia Gu Wen" (Oracle-Bone Scripture), was the earliest evidence of the Chinese use of the written word. These inscriptions revealed that different sicknesses were already named from the problems generated from organs. It was also discovered that wine was already being used externally for medical treatments.(*4)

In the Zhou dynasty (1122-206 B.C.) was recorded a clear classification of four different categories of disorders, which included injuries. The book "Li Ji, Yue Ling Meng Qiu" records treatments for cuts in the skin, muscular swelling, and broken bones, and discussed using both internal and external treatments.

Then, during the Spring and Autumn period (722-481 B.C.), the famous medical book "Nei Jing" discussed in detail the treatment of external injuries and the use of herbs in healing. Massage was the most important part of the treatment.

It was recorded in the Shi Ji (Historical Record) that in the Qing dynasty (255-206 B.C.), the famous doctor Bian Que asked his assistant Zi You to massage Crown Prince Guo, who suffered from epilepsy.

During the Han dynasty (206 B.C.-221 A.D.), the famous doctor Hua Tuo used acupuncture, herbs, and manual therapies (i.e., massage and alignment techniques for dislocated and broken bones). Hua Tuo was the first doctor to emphasize combining acupuncture and massage. Also, Dr. Zhang Ji-Zuo in his book "Shang Han Ran Bing Lun" (The Theory of Typhus Contamination) not only summarized a theoretical and systematic discussion of medical theory, treatments, and diagnosis, but also recorded many methods of massage treatment.

It was recorded in "Han Shu Yi Wen Zhi" (Han's Book of Arts and Scholarship)(206 B.C.-221 A.D.) that "during the reign of the Yellow Emperor, Qi Bo has written ten classics of An Mo....." (*8, *9). Unfortunately, this book has been lost. However, we can see from this mention that An Mo was already being comprehensively studied and practiced. Also in the same period, Dr. Zhang Zhong-Jing in his book "Jin Kui Yao Lue" (Prescriptions from the Golden Chamber) mentioned first aid techniques for someone who had been hanged. He says, "Use the hand to press on the chest, and move frequently."(*10, *11) This is the earliest record of using massage for emergency care.

The oldest Chinese medical book, Huang Di Nei Jing (Internal Classic of the Yellow Emperor) mentions massage. For example, in the "Su Wen" section, the "Xue Qi Xing Zhi Pian" (Chapter on Blood, Qi, Shape, and Spirit), it says: "The pattern frequently gets shocked, and the Jing (i.e., primary Qi channels) and Luo (i.e., smaller channels) are not communicating. Sickness is generated from this lack of feeling. Then cure with An Mo and herbs."(*9, *12) When the systems of the body get shocked often, a pattern of tension builds up and interferes with the Qi and blood circulation. There may be poor communication between the Jing and Luo, or between different Jing channels. When this happens, a part of the body may feel numb. This can be cured with massage and herbs.

Again, in "Yi Fa Fang Yi Lun" (Treatise on Different Methods of Proper Treatment) it says: "In the central area (of China), because the ground is flat and wet, there are therefore millions of living things in the heaven and earth, the food eaten by the people is varied, and the people do not like to work. For this reason, the sicknesses are mostly paralysis and withering, cold and hot. They should be cured by leading (the Qi) with An and Qiao."(*9, *13) When people are inactive, their bodies become insensitive and weak. They are therefore subject to illness caused by rapid changes is the weather. Their condition can be improved by enhancing their Qi circulation through An (i.e., An Mo) and Jiao (i.e., using the feet to massage).

During the Jin dynasty (265-420 A.D.), Dr. Ge Hong in his book: "Shi Hou Jiu Zu Fang" (The Methods of Preparing for Emergencies; Reviving from Unconsciousness) recorded many methods of correcting dislocations, such as of the jaws, and setting broken bones.(*4) This book also says, "To revive from a sudden faint, ..., use the fingers to grab Renzhong cavity, which will immediately revive the patient."(*11, *14) Also, in his book "Bao Pu Zi" Dr. Ge Hong says, "Where there is swelling and pain, using the hands to massage can cure." (*11, *15)

In the Sui dynasty (605-618 A.D.), the book "Sui Shu Bai Guan Zhi" (The Record of Hundreds of Officers in the Sui Dynasty) recorded that in the Imperial Hospital there was a division of An Mo, and there were two An Mo physicians. It was also recorded in Dr. Chao Yuan-Fang's book, "Zhu Bing Yuan Hou Lun" (Thesis on the Origins and Symptoms of Various Diseases) that self-massage for healing was taught in several places.(*9)

By the Tang dynasty (618-907 A.D.), An Mo had become very popular. Old editions of "Tang Shu Zhi Guan Zhi" (Record of Official Positions in the Tang Dynasty) recorded the names of men who were "Masters of An Mo." The new edition of "Record of Official Positions in the Tang Dynasty" had a record of a medical division which had one Doctor of An Mo and four Masters of An Mo.

"Tang Liu Dian" (Tang's Six Records) recorded even more details. It records that there were 56 An Mo technicians and 15 An Mo students in the Imperial Hospital. This was more than the number of acupuncturists and herbalists at that time. This indicates the importance of An Mo in the medical system of that time.

Also in this period, Dr. Wang Tao in his book "Wai Tai Mi Yao" (The Extra Important Secret) mentioned how to use massage to cure stomach pain, saying: "Rub both hands to make them warm, use them to massage the stomach; (this is) able to lead Qi downward."(*11, *16) In addition, Dr. Sun Shi-Mao in his book "Qian Jin Fang" (Thousand Gold Prescriptions) introduced a massage system called Lao Zi's 49 Massage Techniques. In addition, Dr. Lan Dao-Ren's book: "Xian Shou Li Shang Xu Duan Mi Fang" (The Secret Prescriptions for Connecting Broken Bones) further contributed an in-depth theory and methods of treatment for injuries.(*4) In the period of Tang Tian Bao (742-756 A.D.), massage techniques were exported into Japan.(*9) They were the ancestors of today's Japanese massage.

During the Song dynasty (960-1206 A.D.), Dr. Zhang Ben in his book "Yi Shuo" (Talks on Medicine) introduced massage techniques using the feet to increase Qi and blood circulation to expedite the healing of broken bones.(*4) Dr. Pan An-Shi taught how to use massage to help in childbirth.(*11) The fourth volume of "Jing Ji Zong Lun" (The Total Record of Economics) talks about healing, and includes a detailed analysis of how to use An Mo for healing. It says, "(For some sicknesses) you can use An, (for others) use Mo, sometimes use both, all called An Mo. When An (press), do not Mo (rub), (when) Mo (rub), do not An (press). Press with hands, when rubbing, use herbs sometimes. These are An and Mo. Fit (them) to the right purpose."(*11, *17) The book "Ru Men Shi Shi" (The Confucian Point of View) also mentions how massage can increase perspiration, which gave the people a clear idea of how to cure sickness with An Mo.(*11)

In the Yuan dynasty (1206-1368 A.D.), "bone correction" was established as the thirteenth category in the medical system, and became an important part of medical expertise. Tui Na An Mo was a part of bone correction technique. A famous document from this period was Dr. Wei Yi-Lin's "Shi Yi De Xiao Fang" (Effective Prescriptions of Well-known Doctors), which systematically compiled effective prescriptions discovered before the Yuan Dynasty. Dr. Li Zhong-Nan's "Yong Lei Qian Fang" (Permanent Seal Techniques) was another well-known book which discussed bone setting, especially how to correct the bones.(*4)

In the Ming dynasty (1368-1644 A.D.), An Mo was one of the thirteen specialties in the imperial examination. During this period, many more books were published about the treatment of injuries. For example, Dr. Zu Xiou's "Pu Ji Fang, Ze Shang Men" (General Saving Methods, Category for Broken Bones and Injuries), Dr. Wang Ken-Tang's "Yang Yi Zhun Sheng" (The Rules of Healing Injuries) are two of the many publications dealing with the treatment of injuries.(*4) In addition, the book "Xiao Er An Mo Jing" (Massage Classic for Small Children) and the book "Xiao Er Tui Na Mi Jue" (The Secret of Tui Na for Small Children) were also published during this period.(*11) You can see that Tui Na massage had gradually come to be used for treating children's illnesses.

During the Ming and Qing dynasties (1368-1911 A.D.), Tui Na massage became more popular for treating sickness in small children. Acupuncture needs the cooperation of the patient, who must remain still during the treatment. Small children cannot be relied upon to lie still for any length of time, and their movements can break or bend the needles. Tui Na massage requires no needles, and although it is not quite as effective as acupuncture in many cases, it has proven to be safer and easier.

The available documents show that "Xiao Er Tui Na" (Small Children Tui Na) had become one of the main courses of study during this period. For example, during the Ming dynasty, the appendix of Dr. Yang Ji-Zhou's book "Zhen Jiu Da Cheng" (The Great Compendium of Acupuncture and Moxibustion) contained a section entitled "Bao Ying Shen Shu An Mo Jing" (The Classic of Marvelous Massage Techniques for Protecting Babies) which discussed the use of massage to cure sickness of small babies. Also in the same period, Dr. Hu Lian-Bi's book "Xiao Er Tui Na Fang Mai Huo Ying Mi Zhi Quan Shu" (The Complete Book of Secret Keys to Massaging Small Children) and Dr. Zhou Yu-Fu's book "Xiao Er Tui Na Mi Jue" (The Secret of Tui Na for Small Children) also contributed a great deal of knowledge.(*9)

During the Qing dynasty (1644-1911 A.D.), Dr. Cheng Qian's book "Yi Zong Jin Jian; Zheng Gu Xin Fa Yao Zhi" (The Gold Study of Medicine, The Important Keys to Correcting Bones) systematically compiled all of the publications on the subject, and became the most systematic and thorough book on the treatment of injuries. In this book, Dr. Chen divided all of the treatment techniques into eight categories. They are Mo (touch), Jie (connect), Duan (hold up), Ti (lift), Tui (push), Na (grab), An (press), and Mo (rub). In addition to Dr. Chen's book, Dr. Qian Xiu-Chang's "Shang Ke Bu Yao" (The Complementary Important Keys to Treating Injuries), Dr. Gu Shi-Cheng's "Yang Yi Da Quan" (The Great Achievement of Treating Injuries), Hu Ting-Guang's "Shang Ke Hui Cuan" (The Compilation of Injury Categories), Yue Zhu-Quan's "Shang Ke Da Cheng" (The Great Achievement of Injury Categories), all had very systematic and detailed methods for the treatment of injuries.(*4)

During the late Qing dynasty, the use of Tui Na to treat small children had developed even further, and the techniques had even spread to lay society. This is indicated by the countless numbers of books published at this time. Some of the famous ones are Dr. Xiong Ying-Xiong's "Tui Na Guang Yi" (The Wide Definition of Tui Na), Xia Yu-Zhu's "You Ke Tie Jing" (The Iron Mirror for Small Children), and Dr. Luo Qian-An's "You Ke Tui Na Mi Shu" (The Secret Book of Tui Na for Small Children).(*9)

From the Qing dynasty until now, in addition to continuing to practice the massage techniques which had already been developed, a great emphasis began to be placed on Qi massage (also called Qigong healing). Interest in Qi massage has steadily grown, as modern communication speeds word of its effectiveness around the world. This is an exciting period in which traditional medicine must accept the scrutiny of modern science. People today are not satisfied with just getting good results, they also want to know how and why something works.

You can see from this brief account that most of the contributions came from within the medical community. It was not until the beginning of this century that the massage techniques used by martial artists were revealed to lay society. Among the many martial styles of massage, Shaolin Massage was the best known. Shaolin massage focused on physical massage until the practitioner had achieved a high level of understanding of Qi, and then he was introduced to Qi massage. This was very different from the massage which was passed down on Wudang mountain, wherein Qi was always the first concern. On Wudang mountain, the concept of Qi was taught in the very beginning of the training. The Shaolin and the Wudang schools of massage were best known in China for cavity press massage, which is related to the cavity press striking used in the martial arts.

There are other martial styles which have revealed their massage techniques, including "Ying Zhua Men" (Eagle Claw Style), "Qian Long Men" (Heavenly Dragon Style), "Feng Yang Men" (Phoenix Sun Style), "Mi Zong" (Tibetan Secret Style), "Shen Long" (Spiritual Dragon Style), and "Yun Zhan" (Cloud Cutting Style). Some of these styles are derived from Shaolin and Wudang styles. Many of the techniques passed down in these martial styles have been compiled and published, and are now widely available.

1-5. About This Book

This chapter should have given you a basic understanding of the general concepts of Chinese Qigong massage, and of the important role it has played in the history of Chinese medicine. It is important that we now investigate how much of this treasure of knowledge and experience can be borrowed and applied to contemporary and even future medical science. This is the reason I wrote this book. Hopefully, this work will build a bridge to facilitate communication between the East and the West.

Before you read any further, I would like to stress a few points. First, I do not consider that I am an expert in all forms of Chinese Qigong massage. In fact, since the field is so wide and so deep, there are very few people today who can claim to be experts in all aspects of Chinese massage. Therefore, you should not treat this book as an authority. This book is just like many other massage books which can contribute some oriental concepts, and which you can use for reference and to stimulate your thinking. As I explained in the preface, this book is based on my limited knowledge and experience, and on a dozen printed books which discuss Qigong massage in depth. I sincerely hope that those who are masters of Qigong massage will open their minds and hearts, and share their knowledge and experience. This is the only way that Qigong massage can grow and progress today, and it is the only way that this art can gain the widespread respect it deserves.

The second point I would like to emphasize is that in order to learn from the past, we must first remain humble and appreciate the treasure which has been passed to us. Only then will we have the correct attitude for evaluating its value today and in the future.

The science of Chinese Qigong sprang from the natural human reaction to the threat of disease. Like acupuncture, Qigong massage developed out of the basic theory of Qi and its relationship to our health. It is based upon more than five thousand years of practice, as well as a solid theoretical foundation.

If we look at today's medical science, on the one hand, we understand the physical body extremely well. On the other hand, our understanding of Qi or bioelectricity is still in its infancy. It is now beginning to be understood that, if we can thoroughly understand both the physical side and the inner energy side of the human body, medicine can advance to a new stage. It is therefore especially crucial to understand that the information which has been passed down to us may be the gate which leads us to this new field of understanding.

The third point which I would like to make is that when you practice any Qigong, you must first ask: What, Why, and How. "What" means: "What am I looking for?" "What do I expect?" and "What should I do?" Then you must ask, "Why do I need it?" "Why does it work?" "Why must I do it this way instead of that way?." Finally, you must determine, "How does it work?" "How much have I advanced toward my goal?" And "How will I be able to advance further?"

It is very important to understand what you are practicing, not just automatically to repeat what you have learned. Understanding is the root of any work. With understanding you will be able to know your goal. Once you know your goal, your mind can be firm and steady. With this understanding, you will be able to see why something has happened, and what the principles and theories behind it are. Without all of this, your work will be done blindly, and it will be a long and painful process. Only when you are sure what your target is and why you need to reach it should you raise the question of how you are going to accomplish it. The answers to all of these questions form the root of your practice, and will help you to avoid the doubt and confusion that uncertainty brings. If you keep this root, you will be able to apply the theory and make it grow - you will know how to create. Without this root, what you learn will be only branches and flowers, and in time they will wither.

Finally, I would like to make a very important point: The best way to reach a high level of ability and understanding of massage is by doing a great deal of massage. While this book will offer you a general guideline, massaging people is what will give you experience, encourage you to ponder, to continue studying, and to develop yourself. The more you massage yourself and others, the more you will be able to understand. If you wish to advance to the higher levels of ability, it is also advisable to study the basic theory of Chinese medicine. Studying Qigong is also necessary if you wish to understand Qi massage and Qi healing.

Again, I would like to remind you to keep your mind open. If you can do this, you will be more able to see and more willing to accept knowledge from a wide variety of sources. A wise man never stops learning.

References

(*1). "Life's Invisible Current" by Albert L. Huebner, East West Journal, June 1986.

(*2). "The Body Electric" by Robert O. Becker, M.D. and Gary Selden, Quill, William Morrow, New York, 1985.

(*3). "Healing with Nature's Energy" by Richard Leviton, East West Journal, June 1986.

(*4). "中醫骨傷科基礎", 丁繼華, 吳誠德. (The Foundation of the Chinese Medicine in Category of Bone Injury), by Ding Ji-Hua and Wu Chengde, Taipei, Taiwan, 1986.

(*5). 山海經, 東山經："高氏之山, 其上多玉, 其下多箴石."

(*6). 世郭璞："箴石, 可以爲砭針治痛腫者."

(*7). 許慎（説文解字）："砭, 以石刺病也."

(*8). 漢書藝文志："黃帝時歧伯著按摩十卷."

(*9). "按摩大全" 蕭文忠等編. (The Completeness of An Mo), by Xiao Wen-Zhong, etc., Taipei, Taiwan, 1986.

(*10). 張仲景（金匱要略）："以手按據胸上, 數動之."

(*11). "按摩推拿手法萃錦" 李茂林. (The Refined Collection of An Mo Tui Na Techniques), by Li Mao-Lin, Peiking, China, 1985.

(*12). 素問血氣形志篇："形數驚恐, 經絡不通, 病生於不仁, 治之以按摩醪醴藥."

(*13). 異法方宜論："中央者, 其地平以濕, 天地所以生萬物也衆, 其民食雜而不勞, 其病多痿厥寒熱, 其治宜導引按蹻."

(*14). 時後備急方："救卒中惡死, ..., 令爪其病人仁中, 取醒."

(*15). 葛洪（抱朴子）："其腫痛所在, 以摩之皆手下即愈."

(*16). 王燾（外臺秘要）："兩手相摩令熱, 以摩腹, 令氣下."

(*17). 經濟總論："可按可摩, 時兼而用, 通謂之按摩；按之弗摩, 按之以手, 摩或兼以藥, 曰按曰摩, 适所用也."

Chapter 2
General Foundations

2-1. Introduction

In the last chapter, we briefly introduced the general theory of massage. However, in order to massage effectively, you need to have a much deeper understanding of the theory. This, plus the experience you have accumulated, will greatly increase your ability to accurately analyze the needs of the patient. Remember, knowledge is the Yin side of massage, and it forms the foundation for the Yang side, which is practicing massage.

Although the basic theory remains the same in all four categories of Chinese Qigong massage, the goals of each category and the theory of how to approach the goals are often very different. For example, while Tui Na and Dian Xue massage both regulate the Qi levels in the channels, they each go about it in quite different ways. In order to avoid confusion, we will discuss how each category applies the theory when we introduce that category.

In this chapter, we will discuss some of the important concepts which form the foundation for all four categories. However, the most important thing you need to know is the structure of the human body. Lacking this, you will be like a blind man walking in the street.

The first thing you need to know about the physical body is that it is only a part of your entire being. According to Chinese medicine and religion, a living human body consists of three parts: 1. a Yang part, the physical body, which manifests the activities (life) of the body, 2. a Yin part, the inner energy (Qi or bioelectricity) part of the body, which nourishes the physical body and keeps it alive, and 3. the refined product of the Yin and Yang parts: the spiritual or mental body.

Western medicine usually devotes all of its attention to problems in the physical body, and usually ignores problems in the energy body. Because of this, there is a wealth of publications about the structure of the physical body, and the level of understanding is quite profound. It cannot be denied that in the understanding of the physical human body, Western science is the world leader. However, in regards to the structure of the inner energy body, it is still in the beginning stage. In fact, it was not until the last two decades that the concept of bioelectricity was even recognized by Western medicine.

As mentioned in the first chapter, Yin (Qi) is the root of the life while Yang (physical action) is the manifestation of life. Yin and Yang must be balanced. Whenever there is a deficiency or excess in either the Yin side or the Yang side, the body will become sick. Most illnesses are caused by the abnormal distribution and circulation of Qi, i.e., by the Yin side of the body. Therefore, when you study the structure of the human body, you must not limit yourself by studying only the physical side. Both sides are mutually related and cannot be separated. However, you must also beware of going to the other extreme and mixing or confusing the two concepts.

Many people still confuse the Qi distribution system with the nervous system. We know from Western science that physically there are three major networks in the human body: the circulatory system, the nervous system, and the lymphatic system. All three are physical, visible systems. However, in order to keep functioning properly, these three systems need energy, which the Chinese call Qi, and Western science calls bioelectricity. Naturally, in order to supply Qi to these systems efficiently, the Qi system must be organized and structured similarly to the other three systems. Because of this, it is not really surprising that many people still believe that the Qi system is just the Chinese name for the nervous system.

To clear up this confusion, in the next section we will briefly review the physical structure of the human body. If you would like to know about this subject in more detail, there are many anatomy books available. In the third section, we will summarize the structure of the human Qi body. If you would like to know more about this subject, many books on Chinese medicine are now available in English. Then, in the fourth section, we will explain the refined product of the physical and Qi bodies, the spirit or the mental body.

Once you have a clear understanding of the structure of the human body, the fifth section will discuss the "gates" or "junctions" in the body. Understanding the gates or junctions is a crucial key to performing a successful massage. Finally, in the last section, we will list a number of important points to remember that apply to all categories of massage. Naturally, there are also many other rules which apply to one category or the other, but we will bring these up when those categories are discussed.

2-2. Understanding the Physical Body

First, let us take a look at the general structure of the body. When you look at a portion of your body, for example, an arm, the first thing you see is the skin (Figure 2-1). On the skin are hairs and thousands of pores. The pores are like gates through which waste is eliminated from your body, and through which Qi is exchanged with the environment. According to Chinese Qigong, if your Qi is able to

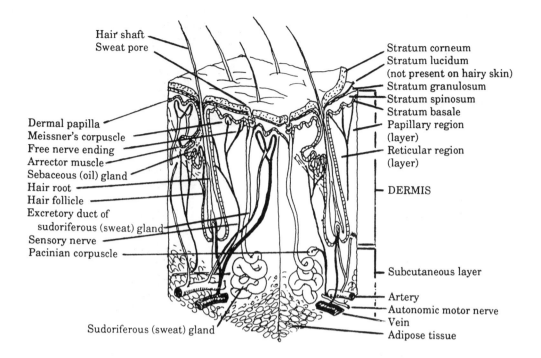

Figure 2-1. Anatomical structure of the skin.

reach the skin and abundantly nourish every cell and the circulatory systems there (i.e., if your Guardian Qi is strong), the skin and hair will stay youthful and healthy. However, when the Qi is weak or the supply is abnormal, which happens, for example, when you grow older, the symptoms appear first in the hair and skin. Therefore, one of the purposes of general massage is to lead Qi to the skin, to improve the smooth circulation of the blood, and to maintain the sensitivity of the nerves.

Right under the surface of the skin is a thick layer of fat. Fat is the stored essence of food. In other words, when we eat more than we need, the excess which is not excreted is stored in the body as fat. This fat is usually carried by the blood cells to every part of the body. The more fat there is in the blood stream, the more sluggish the circulation is. Fat can be stored under the skin, in the fasciae, and on in the bone marrow. The more fat you have stored in your body, the poorer your Qi and blood circulation will be.

Underneath the layer of fat, but before the muscles, is a layer of fascia. Fasciae is found in many places in the body. The first place is between the skin and the muscles, the second place is between the layers of muscle, the third place is between the muscles and the bones, and the last place is around the internal organs. Next time you buy a chicken, if you cut it open and examine it you should be able to locate these fasciae, which are thin layers of transparent membrane. Fat is stored in the fasciae. It is also known that the fat and the fascia are not conductors of Qi. This means whenever the Qi is passing through fasciae, the resistance will be higher and affect

Figure 2-2.
Superficial anatomical structure of the posterior aspect of the arm

Figure 2-3.
Anatomical structure of the middle layer of the anterior aspect of the arm.

the Qi circulation. Therefore, one of the purposes of general massage is to remove the fat accumulated in the fasciae. Physical exercise can also accomplish this.

Between the fasciae and the muscles are found the veins, nerves, and sometimes lymph vessels (Figure 2-2). If you remove some of the muscles, you will see the main arteries, and the main nerves (Figure 2-3). Beneath the muscle is the bone (Figure 2-4), and inside the bone is the marrow (Figure 2-5).

Now let us first look at the body's two physical circulatory systems: the blood vascular system and the lymph vascular system. Then we will review another important system, the nervous system.

1. Blood System:

Blood is considered to be the "elixir of life" in the West. Blood is mainly composed of red cells, white cells, platelets and plasma. The red cells carry nourishment (including oxygen and Qi) to the organs and tissues through the arteries. Waste materials are also carried away from the tissues by the blood to the eliminative organs. The blood finally returns to the heart through the veins. The blood acts as

1. Epiphysis
2. Spongy bone
3. Medullary cavity
4. Compact bone
5. Nutrient foramen
6. Diaphysis

Figure 2-4.
Deep anatomical structure of the anterior aspect of the arm.

Figure 2-5. Bone and bone marrow.

a conduit for essential products made by various organs, carrying these products to other organs which need them to function properly and survive. Each blood cell has properties not unlike that of a small battery, allowing them to store electrical charges and carry them throughout the body. Because of this, blood may also help to equalize the energy level throughout the body, facilitating harmonious interaction between all the diverse bodily components that it supplies.

The main function of white blood cells is to seek out, identify, and destroy germs by literally eating them alive. The white cells are not alone, however, in their germ hunting mission. Other parts of the blood, including its fluid portion (i.e., plasma), carry germ-killing substances. There are proteins in the plasma which play an integral role in this endeavor. Finally, platelets, along with other substances, help to enable the blood to coagulate (i.e., solidify). This avoids major loss of blood from minor cuts or wounds.

There are a number of important points here. The first is that the blood cells are the nourishment conveyors of the body. Any defect in the smooth flow of blood in the blood vessels will be reflected in a failure of the other cells of the body to receive the proper amount of oxygen, nutrition, and Qi. New, fresh blood cells are constantly being produced in the bone marrow to replace the old cells. When the bone marrow is not functioning properly or has been damaged through neglect or old age, the blood cells produced will be of inferior quality. According to Chinese Qigong, if you want the marrow to keep producing healthy blood cells, you have to keep the marrow well-supplied with Qi. This has become a very important part of Chinese Qigong, and is called "Bone Marrow Washing Qigong." If you are interested in more on this subject, please refer to the YMAA book "Muscle/Tendon Changing and Marrow/Brain Washing Chi Kung."

The second important point is that, in order to keep the blood cells supplying the body with nourishment and removing waste, the circulatory system must be healthy. While it is very difficult to use massage to improve the Qi supply to the bone marrow, it is very easy to use general massage to improve blood circulation. The main blood vessels are located under the muscles, between the muscles, and on the surface of the muscles. Since tensing the muscles constricts the blood vessels, massaging the muscles will relieve tension on the vessels and improve circulation. In addition, general massage can help to reduce stored fat, thereby increasing the responsiveness of this vital circulatory system.

2. Lymphatic System:

Lymph is a transparent, watery, colorless or sometimes slightly yellow fluid. The lymphatic system consists of this fluid, the vessels that carry it into the blood - the lymph vessels or lymphatics, and a series of lymph organs including the lymph nodes, tonsils, spleen, and thymus (Figure 2-6).

Lymph vessels of the lymph-capillary type arise in nearly all parts of the body. Lymph-capillaries take up any blood-plasma which has been discharged for nourishment purposes from the blood-capillaries into the tissue-spaces, and returns it into veins near the heart. Most of these lymphatics empty themselves into one main reservoir called the thoracic duct, which runs upward along the anterior of the spine, opening into large veins on the left side of the neck, at its base. The rest of the lymphatics empty into a smaller reservoir which runs into corresponding veins on the right side of the neck base. Lymph's primary function is to remove bacteria and certain proteins from the tissues, to transport fat from the intestines, and to supply lymphocytes to the blood.

Lymph nodes, which are also commonly referred to as lymph glands, are oval or round bodies which are found adjacent to the lymphatic vessels. They supply lymphocytes to the circulatory system and cleanse the lymph by removing bacteria and foreign particles. One commonly known example of these glands are the tonsils.

One of the largest lymphoid structures in the human body is the spleen. The spleen, which filters and stores blood, is located on the left side of the torso below the diaphragm. Finally, the thymus is a ductless glandlike body, positioned just behind the top of the

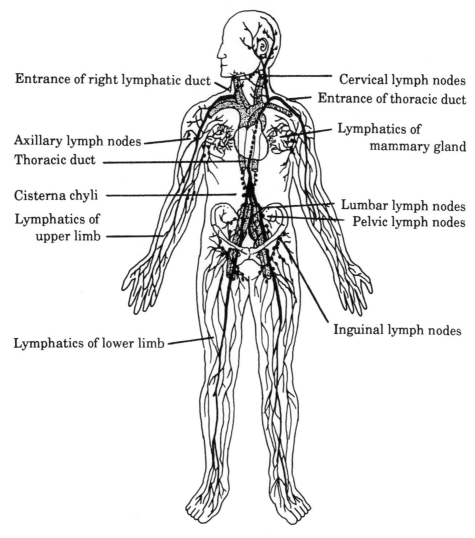

Figure 2-6. Major lymph vessels of the body.

sternum. The thymus reaches its maximum development in child-hood, and plays some part in building resistance to disease. However, by adulthood this organ is usually vestigial, having no further known use.

3.   The Nervous System:

A nerve is a bundle of fibers uniting the central nervous system with the organs and other parts of the body. Nerves relay sensory stimuli as well as motor impulses from different parts of the body to one another.

All multicellular animals except sponges possess nervous systems. They are essentially regulatory mechanisms, controlling internal bodily functions and responses to external stimuli. The human nervous system is made up of two component sub-systems: the central nervous system (CNS) and the peripheral nervous system (PNS)(Figure 2-7).

Figure 2-7. Basic organization of the nervous system.

Making up the central nervous system (CNS) are the brain and the spinal cord, which are contained and protected within the skull and the spine respectively. The CNS integrates, interprets, and transmits messages to and from the brain and the periphery of the body.

Making up the peripheral nervous system (PNS) is all nervous tissue found outside of the skull and spinal column, including not only the nerve fibers that carry impulses, but also groupings of fibers (plexuses) and nerve cell bodies (ganglions) that are found in the periphery. The PNS registers changes in the internal and external environments of the body, transmitting this information to the CNS for action, and then delivering the orders of the CNS to muscles and glands for response.

The PNS includes 12 pairs of cranial nerves which attach to the brain and their associated ganglions, as well as 31 pairs of spinal nerves and their ganglions. Finally, the PNS also includes specialized receptors and endings on muscles.

In terms of the function and interaction of all these constituent components, the PNS is simple yet efficient. It is "built" out of somatic fibers (somatic nervous system) that provide the nerves for the skeletal muscles as well as the skin's special receptors (for touch, pressure, heat, cold), and autonomic fibers (autonomic nervous system). The autonomic fibers carry impulses to smooth and cardiac muscles and glands, and from visceral receptors (Figure 2-8). These fibers make possible the reflexes which control breathing, heart rate, blood pressure, and other bodily functions in an involuntary and unbroken manner. Most organs receive fibers from two subdivisions of the autonomic nervous system. The parasympathetic (craniosacral) division, which is comprised of certain cranial nerves and several of the sacral spinal nerves, furnishes nervous influences for the purpose of conservation of body sources and maintenance of nominal function levels. The sympathetic (thoracolumbar) division, which is comprised of the thoracic and lumber spinal nerves, furnishes impulses for the purpose of elevating body activity in order to tolerate or resist stressful or hazardous situations. In this way an organ may have its operation intensified or diminished according to the demands of the situation for survival.

This brief anatomic discussion of the nervous system shows us that the brain and spinal cord are the center of our feeling and functioning. We have seen that nerves from the spinal cord extend out and connect to the entire body, including the limbs and also the internal organs.

There are a number of other facts about the nervous system that are also important. First, our state of mind is linked to the condition of our physical body through our nervous system. This means that if we are mentally tense or relaxed, our physical body will react accordingly. Second, the nervous system is constructed of tissue fibers, which are part of the material side of our body. In order to function properly, in fact, even to stay alive, this material needs Qi. Third, if we compare the system of Qi distribution with the nervous system we see that, although they are related, they are not the same

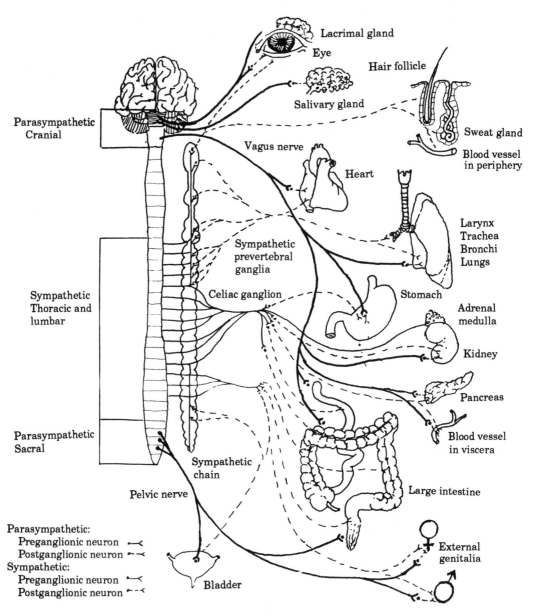

Figure 2-8. A schematic representation of the autonomic nervous
system and the organs it serves.

system. The Qi circulatory system does not supply Qi only to the
nervous system exclusively, it supplies it to all of the body's cells.

The nervous system plays a critical role in the practice of
Qigong. The nervous system enables us to feel what is going on
everywhere in our body. Since the mind leads the Qi, if we want to
lead Qi somewhere we have to be able to feel that place. If we cannot
feel that place, then the mind cannot lead the Qi there, since it does
not know where it is.

The nervous system is responsible for our ability to feel, and it is
our ability to feel that governs the Qi. This means that the condition
of the nervous system is directly related to the Qi circulation in our
body. In Qigong massage therefore, while we should pay particular

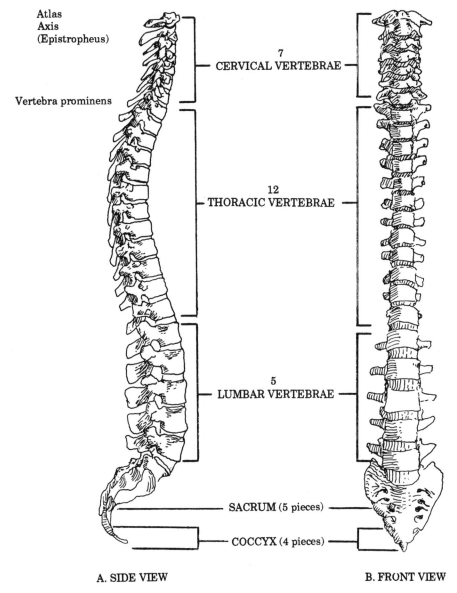

Figure 2-9. Side and front views of the vertebral column.

attention to the Qi system, the nervous system should be second in our priorities.

To massage the nervous system, you start with the central nervous system, which includes the brain and the spinal cord, and then you loosen up the places where the peripheral nervous system extends out from the spinal cord to the limbs and internal organs. All of these junctions are located on the sides of the vertebrae.

After the head, the spine is the most important place to massage. The spine consists of seven cervical vertebrae (the neck), twelve thoracic vertebrae (the rib area), five lumbar vertebrae (the waist area), the sacrum (which consists of five pieces), and the coccyx or tailbone (four pieces)(Figure 2-9).

It is important to know how the central nervous system relates to the internal organs, which was illustrated in Figure 2-8. Massaging the nervous system in and around the spine stimulates the corresponding internal organs and improves their functioning. This means that when you massage the spine, you indirectly massage the internal organs.

Finally, you also need to know how the central nervous system is related to the skin on the limbs. Since you touch a person's skin when you do general massage, and since sections of the skin are related to sections of the central nervous system, you can smooth out the Qi and relieve nervous tension from the spine to the ends of the limbs. An area of the skin with sensory fibers from a single spinal nerve is called a dermatome. Figure 2-10 shows the dermatomes of the arms and legs.

2-3. Understanding the Qi Body

Before discussing the Qi body, I would first like you to understand that you cannot actually see the Qi circulatory system. This is because we cannot see the difference between regular muscle tissue and the electrically conductive fascial tissue with the naked eye. At present, it seems reasonable to conclude that all of the Qi channels are hidden in these tissues. Exactly how these channels are formed is a mystery that is still awaiting further study with modern equipment. Next, in order to help you understand the Qi circulatory system, I would like to review some of the important concepts in Chinese medicine. This will help you to understand the rest of this section.

Qi:

Although we discussed the definition of Qi in the last chapter, it is so important that it is worth going over again. Qi is the energy which circulates within the body. Your entire body is like a factory and your organs are like the many machines operating inside the factory. Your brain is like management, directing the entire operation. In order to keep the factory functioning properly, you need a power supply. The power supply is connected to each machine with many wires and cables. Each machine must receive the appropriate level of power; too much power will damage the machine and shorten its life, and too little power will not enable the machine to function properly. You can see that without a proper power supply in the factory, production will be off, and if the power supply stops, the entire factory is dead. It is the same with your body. When your body does not have a normal energy (Qi) supply, the organs will not function properly, and you will become sick; and if the Qi circulation stops, you will die.

You should realize that your entire body is alive, including every blood cell, every nerve tissue, and every muscle fiber. All of these physical, fundamental structures of the body need Qi to maintain

Figure 2-10. Dermatomes of the arms and legs.

their existence and their ability to function. The system which distributes Qi throughout your body is much like the wiring system in a factory, connecting the power source to the machines.

From the viewpoint of function, Chinese medical science classifies Qi in the following ways:

1. **Organ Qi:** This Qi is responsible for the functioning of the organs.
2. **Channel Qi:** This Qi is responsible for the transportive and moving functions of the channels.
3. **Nourishing Qi:** The main responsibilities of this Qi are trans-

Figure 2-11. The Shanzhong cavity (Co-17).

forming and creating blood. Nourishing Qi also moves with the blood and helps the blood to nourish the tissues of the body.

4. **Guardian Qi:** (Also commonly translated as Protective Qi). This Qi circulates outside the channels and the organs. Guardian Qi's responsibilities are to warm the organs, to travel between the skin and the flesh to regulate the opening and closing of the pores, and to protect and moisten the skin, hair, and nails. This Qi is able to provide the body with a defense against external negative influences such as cold weather.

5. **Ancestral Qi:** This Qi gathers (resides) in the chest with its center at the Shanzhong cavity (Co-17)(Figure 2-11). Ancestral Qi is able to travel up to the throat and down to the abdomen. It is responsible for breathing and speaking, regulating heart beat, and, when cultivated through meditation, Ancestral Qi can strengthen the body.

	WOOD 木	FIRE 火	EARTH 土	METAL 金	WATER 水
Direction	East	South	Center	West	North
Season	Spring	Summer	Long Summer	Autumn	Winter
Climatic Condition	Wind	Summer Heat	Dampness	Dryness	Cold
Process	Birth	Growth	Transformation	Harvest	Storage
Color	Green	Red	Yellow	White	Black
Taste	Sour	Bitter	Sweet	Pungent	Salty
Smell	Goatish	Burning	Fragrant	Rank	Rotten
Yin Organ	Liver	Heart	Spleen	Lungs	Kidneys
Yang Organ	Gall Bladder	Small Intestine	Stomach	Large Intestine	Bladder
Opening	Eyes	Tongue	Mouth	Nose	Ears
Tissue	Sinews	Blood Vessels	Flesh	Skin/Hair	Bones
Emotion	Anger	Happiness	Pensiveness	Sadness	Fear
Human Sound	Shout	Laughter	Song	Weeping	Groan

Table 2-1. Table of Correspondences associated with the Five Phases.

Blood:

The Western concept of blood is only part of the Chinese conception of blood. Although blood is seen as a red fluid, in Chinese medical science it is also regarded as a force which is involved with the sensitivity of the sense organs and the inner vitality of the body. Since the main responsibility of blood is to carry nourishment to every part of the body, it is closely related to Nourishing Qi.

Qi and Blood:

In Chinese medicine, Qi is considered Yang and blood is considered Yin. Qi is said to be the "commander" of blood because blood relies on Qi for its generation (out of food and air), and for its power to move through and remain in the blood vessels. It is also said that blood is the "mother" of Qi because the strength of Qi depends upon the nutrition and moisture carried in the blood. Therefore, Qi and blood are believed to complement each other.

Organs (Viscera):

The concept of the organs in Chinese medicine differs significantly from that of Western medicine. In Chinese medicine the organs are systems of functions, and not mere physical objects. Generally, this means that within the description of the organs, almost all of the body's functions can be defined and explained.

In Chinese medical science, the organs are divided into two main groups: the Yin (Inner) organs and Yang (Outer) organs. There are six Yin organs and six Yang organs. Five of the Yin organs (excluding the pericardium) are called "Zang," which means viscera. These five (liver, heart, spleen, lungs, and kidneys) are considered the core of the entire system. Usually, when a discussion involves the channels and all the organs, the pericardium is added; otherwise it is treated as an adjunct of the heart. According to Chinese medicine, the Yin organs "store and do not drain." That means that their functions are directed toward sustaining homeostasis, both physically and mentally.

The six Yang organs are called "Fu," which means 'bowels,' and include the gall bladder, small intestine, large intestine, stomach, bladder, and triple burner. According to Chinese medicine, these Yang organs "drain and do not store." This refers to their responsibility in the transformation and the disposal of food and waste. All the Yang organs receive food or a product of food, and then pass it along.

In Table 2-1, you will notice that each Yang organ is associated with a Yin organ by a special Yin/Yang relationship (or Inner/Outer relationship). Pairs of related Yin and Yang organs belong to the same Phase, and their Qi channels are sequential to each other in Qi circulation. They are so closely linked that a disease in one will usually affect the other.

Yin and Yang:

Yin and Yang are not contradictory. Nor is one considered "good," and the other "bad." To obtain health, a harmony is sought between them and any imbalance is avoided. Yin and Yang are relative, not absolute.

Five Phases (Five Elements)(Wu Xing):

The five phases are Wood, Fire, Earth, Metal, and Water. They are also commonly translated as the "Five Elements." In Chinese, Xing means to walk or to move; probably more pertinent, it means a process. The Five Phases are thought of as the five properties inherent in all things. Each phase symbolizes a category of related functions and qualities. For example, Wood is linked with active functions that are in phase with growth or with increasing. Fire expresses that the functions have reached a maximum state and are ready to decline. Metal represents declining functions. Water symbolizes that the functions have declined and are ready to grow. And finally, Earth is associated with balance or neutrality. Therefore, Earth is the center point of the five phases.

The relationships between the five phases are shown in Figure 2-12.

Qi Channels and Vessels:

"Jing" is commonly translated "meridians" or "primary Qi channels." Your body has twelve channels, which Chinese medicine considers to be like rivers of Qi. Each channel, although referred to in the singular, is actually a pair of mirror-image channels, one on either side of the body. One end of each of these twelve channels is associated with one of the twelve organs, while the other end is connected to a toe or finger (six channels are connected to the fingers and the other six are connected to the toes).

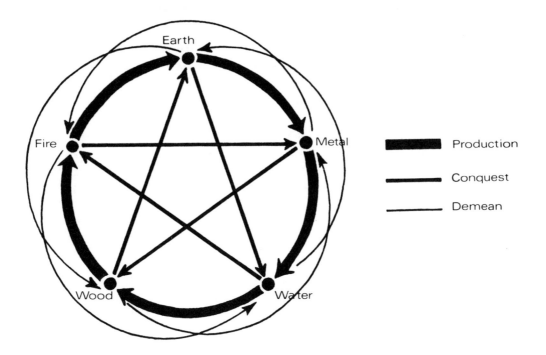

Figure 2-12. Relationships between the Five Phases.

There are eight "Qi Mai" or "Qi vessels" in your body. They are often compared to reservoirs because they store Qi for your system. They can also be compared to batteries and capacitors in an electrical system. Batteries store and then release electrical current, and capacitors regulate the electrical current in the same way that the vessels regulate the Qi in your channels and organs.

There are other Qi channels called "Luo" or "Qi branches." There are millions of Luo spreading out from the channels to distribute Qi to every cell in the body. The Luo carry Qi from the channels outward to nourish the skin, hair, eyes, nails, etc., and also inward to the bone marrow to maintain the production of blood cells. Luo also connect the organs, enabling them to communicate and cooperate with each other.

The next term you must know is "Xue," which is translated as "cavity." Your body has more than seven hundred of these cavities, through which acupuncturists access the Qi channels with needles or other methods.

In order for you to be healthy, the Qi must flow smoothly and continuously in the channels. However, sometimes there are blockages, and the flow becomes stagnant. Blockages can be caused by eating poor quality food, by injuries, or by the physical degeneration that occurs as you age. Another problem occurs when the Qi is not flowing at the proper level. Acupuncturists have several ways of treating these problems, including the insertion of needles in certain cavities to adjust the flow of Qi.

The Twelve Primary Qi Channels

In this subsection we will briefly review the twelve primary Qi channels. As a Qigong masseur you need to know how the Qi in each channel and related organ can be affected by the seasons, the weather, emotions, and food. Table 2-1 offers you a guideline to these relationships.

You should also know the organ's Yin and Yang. In our body, there are six Yang organs and six Yin organs. Each Yang organ is associated with a Yin organ by a special Yin/Yang relationship. Paired Yin and Yang organs belong to the same phase in the Five Phases. Their channels are sequential to each other in the circulation of Qi, their functions are closely related, and disease in one usually affects the other. In Chinese medicine, the channel corresponding to the Yang organ is often used to treat disorders of its related Yin organ.

In the limbs, the Yang channels are on the external side of the limbs while the Yin channels are on the internal side. Generally speaking, the outsides of the limbs are more Yang and are more resistant and prepared for an attack, while the internal sides are more Yin and weaker.

The organs are further subdivided in order to distinguish the different levels of the Yin/Yang characteristics. The Yang organs are divided into Greater Yang (Taiyang), Lesser Yang (Shaoyang), and Yang Brightness (Yangming). The Yin organs are divided into Greater Yin (Taiyin), Lesser Yin (Shaoyin), and Absolute Yin (Jueyin). In the following discussion, all of the classifications will be shown in the title, for example: the Lung Channel of Hand — Greater Yin.

1. **The Lung Channel of Hand — Greater Yin** (Figure 2-13)
A. **Course:**
    Course #1:
    (1). Stomach (Zhong Jiao, middle triple burner) - (2). Large intestine - (3). Diaphragm - (4). Lung - (5). Throat - (6). Upper Arm - (7). Mid-Elbow - (8). Forearm - (9). Wrist - (10). Thenar - (11). Pollex (Shaoshang, L-11).
    Course #2:
    (12). Above the styloid process at the wrist - (13). Index Finger (Shangyang, LI-1).

B. **Related Viscera:**
    Lung (Pertaining Organ), large intestine, stomach, and kidney.

C. **Cavities:**
    Zhongfu (L-1), Yunmen (L-2), Tianfu (L-3), Xiabai (L-4), Qize (L-5), Kongzui (L-6), Lieque (L-7), Jingqu (L-8), Taiyuan (L-9), Yuji (L-10), and Shaoshang (L-11).

D. **Discussion:**

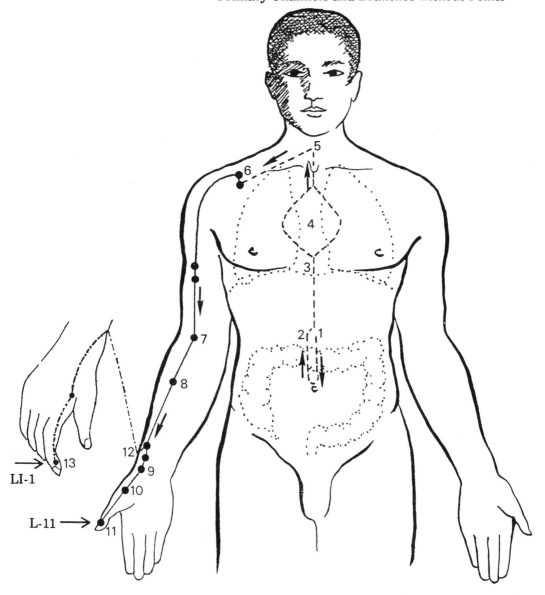

Figure 2-13. The Lung Channel of the Hand-Greater Yin.

The lungs (Yin) and the large intestine (Yang) are considered paired organs. From Table 2-1 you can see that they belong to Metal in the Five Phases, the westerly direction, the season of autumn, the dry climatic condition, the color white, the pungent taste, the rank odor, the emotion of sadness, and the sound of weeping. Their opening is the nose, and they govern skin and hair.

In Qigong practice, since the lungs belong to Metal, they are able to regulate heartburn. The heart belongs to Fire. Whenever the heart has excess Qi, deep breathing is able to lead the heart's fire to the lungs, and therefore cool the heartburn. When the weather is changing from damp, hot summer into dry and cool autumn, lungs are the first organ to sense the change. If your lungs are not able to readjust themselves to fit the new situation smoothly, you will catch a cold. The lungs access the outside world through your nose. The lungs are responsible for taking Qi from the air, and for the energy (Qi) state of the body.

Breathing is considered a strategy for leading Qi to the extremities such as skin and hair. When your breathing is regulated properly, you are able to strengthen your body's Guardian Qi and generate an expansive Qi shield to protect your body. You are also able to raise or lower your Qi state through your breathing. For example, when you are angry, deep breathing is able to calm your excited Qi state.

The lungs are sensitive to emotional changes, especially when you are sad or angry. They also control that part of the liquid metabolism which distributes liquid to the skin.

Because the lungs are usually the first to be attacked by exogenous diseases, they are called the Delicate Organ. These diseases can also cause what is called the Non-Spreading of the Lung Qi. The main symptom of a problem with the lungs is coughing, which is a form of Rebellious Qi (since the lung Qi normally flows downward). If coughing is also accompanied by lassitude, shortness of breath, light foamy phlegm, and weakness in the voice, it is called Deficient Lung Qi. However, if the cough is a dry one, with little phlegm, a parched throat and mouth, and Deficient Yin symptoms (such as night sweating, low grade fever, red cheeks, etc.), the condition is referred as Deficient Lung Yin.

2. The Large Intestine Channel of Hand - Yang Brightness
(Figure 2-14)

A. Course:

Course #1:

(1). Index finger (Shangyang, LI-1) - (2). Wrist - (3). Elbow - (4). Shoulder Joint - (5). Governing vessel at Dazhui (Gv-14) - (6). Supraclavicular Fossa (Quepen, S-12) - (7). Lung - (8). Diaphragm - (9). Large intestine.

Course #2:

(6). Supraclavicular fossa - (10). Neck - (11). Cheek - (12). Lower Gum - (13). Renzhong (Gv-26) - (14). Side of the nose (Yingxiang, LI-20).

B. Related Viscera:

Large intestine (Pertaining Organ), lung, and stomach.

C. Cavities:

Shangyang (LI-1), Erjian (LI-2), Sanjian (LI-3), Hegu (LI-4), Yangxi (LI-5), Pianli (LI-6), Wenliu (LI-7), Xianlian (LI-8), Shanglian (LI-9), Shousanli (LI-10), Quchi (LI-11), Zhouliao (LI-12), Hand-Wuli (LI-13), Binao (LI-14), Jianyu (LI-15), Jugu (LI-16), Tianding (LI-17), Futu (LI-18), Heliao (LI-19), and Yingxiang (LI-20).

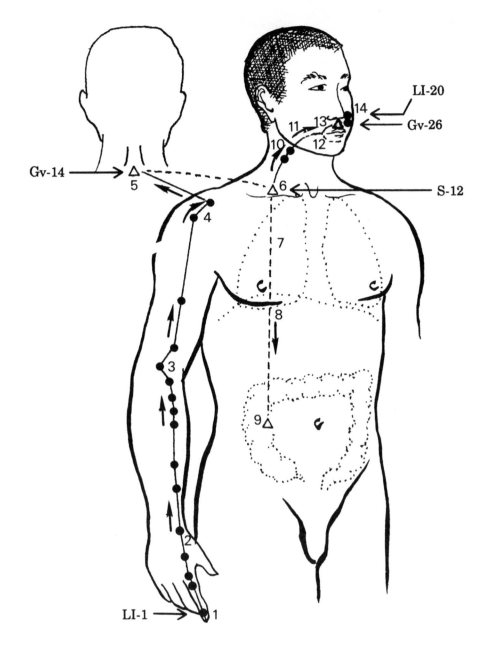

Figure 2-14. The Large Intestine Channel of the Hand-Yang Brightness.

D. Discussion:

The lungs (Yin) and the large intestine (Yang) are considered paired organs. From Table 2-1 you can see that they belong to Metal in the Five Phases, the westerly direction, the season of autumn, the dry climatic condition, the color white, the pungent taste, the rank odor, the emotion of sadness, and the sound of weeping. Their opening is the nose, and they govern skin and hair.

The main function of the large intestine is the metabolism of water and the passing of water. It extracts water from the waste material received from the small intestine, sends it on to the urinary bladder, and excretes the solid material as stool. Many disorders affecting this organ are categorized as spleen and stomach patterns. Certain abdominal pains are considered manifestations of a blockage of Qi or blood in the large intestine.

In Qigong, the Dan Tian in the lower abdomen is considered the residence of Original Qi. In order to keep this Qi at its residence, this area must be strong and healthy. The Qi circulating around the intestines must not be stagnant. When you practice Qigong you must learn how to regulate your breathing to smooth the Qi flow in the large intestine and the lungs. This will allow you to relax the front of your body and regulate the Qi flow in the other organs.

3.   The Stomach Channel of Foot - Yang Brightness (Figure 2-15)

A. Course:

Course #1:

(1). Sides of the nose (Yingxiang, LI-20) - (2). Root of the nose - (3). Lateral side of the nose - (4). Upper gum - (5). Renzhong (Gv-26) - (6). Chengjiang (Co-24) - (7). Daying (S-5) - (8). Jiache (S-6) - (9). Ear - (10). Hair line - (11). Shenting (Gv-24).

Course #2:

(7). Daying (S-5) - (12). Renying (S-9) - (13). Throat - (14). Into the chest - (15). Through the diaphragm to Zhongwan (Co-12).

Course #3:

(16). Infraclavicular fossa - (17). Along the sides of the umbilicus - (18). Qichong (S-30). - (19). Biguan (S-31) - (20). Futu (S-32) - (21). Dubi (S-35) - (22). Lateral side of tibia - (23). Dorsal aspect of the foot - (24). Lateral side of the tip of the second toe (Lidui, S-45).

Course #4:

(25). Below the knee - (26). Lateral side of the middle toe.

Course #5:

(27). Dorsum of the foot (Chongyang, S-42) - (28). Along the medial margin of the hallus and emerges out at its tip (Yinbai, Sp-1).

B.   Related Viscera:

Stomach (Pertaining Organ), spleen, heart, small intestine, and large intestine.

C.   Cavities:

Chengqi (S-1), Sibai (S-2), Juliao (S-3), Dicang (S-4), Daying (S-5), Jiache (S-6), Xiaguan (S-7), Touwei (S-8), Renying (S-9), Shuitu (S-10), Qishe (S-11), Quepen (S-12), Qihu (S-13), Kufang (S-14), Wuyi (S-15), Yingchuang (S-16), Ruzhong (S-17), Rugen (S-18), Burong (S-19), Chengman (S-21), Liangmen (S-21), Guanmen (S-22), Taiyi (S-23), Huaroumen (S-24), Tianshu (S-25), Wailing (S-26), Daju (S-27), Shuidao (S-28), Guilai (S-29), Qichong (S-30), Biguan (S-31), Futu (S-32), Yinshi (S-33), Liangqiu (S-34), Dubi (S-35), Zusanli (S-36), Shangjuxu (S-37), Tiaokou (S-38), Xiajuxu (S-39), Fenglong (S-40), Jiexi (S-41), Chongyang (S-42), Xiangu (S-43), Neiting (S-44), Lidui (S-45).

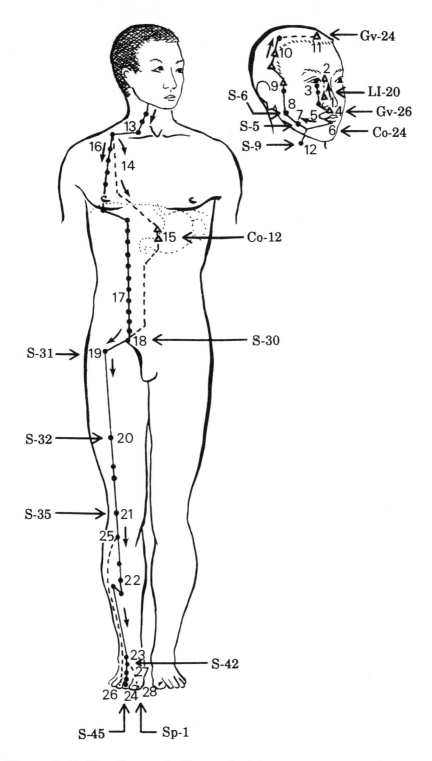

Figure 2-15. The Stomach Channel of the Foot-Yang Brightness.

D. Discussion:

The spleen (Yin) and the stomach (Yang) are paired organs. They belong to Earth in the Five Phases, the center, the season of long summer (the end of summer), the climatic condition of dampness, the color yellow, the emotion of pensiveness, the taste of sweetness, fragrant odor, and the sound of singing. Their opening is the mouth and they control the flesh and the limbs.

The Yin/Yang relationship between the spleen and the stomach is a particularly strong example of the relationship between organs. The stomach receives food while the spleen transports nutrients. The stomach moves things downward while the spleen moves things upward. The stomach likes dampness while the spleen likes dryness.

Though there are some patterns relating to deficiency of the stomach (many of these originate in the spleen), most stomach disorders are caused from excess. Stomach Fire gives a painful, burning sensation in the stomach, unusual hunger, bleeding of the gums, constipation, and halitosis.

Once saliva has begun the process of digestion, food passes to the stomach, located in the middle Sanjiao (middle triple burner) area. The stomach breaks down the food, and then passes it on to the intestines, where the essence is absorbed and converted into Qi, and circulated through the entire body.

The stomach is related to the emotion of pensiveness. When you are upset, the stomach will not function normally. In Qigong, regulating the mind is the first step to maintaining the stomach in a healthy condition. The type of food you eat is the second consideration. The proper amount and quality of food will help you to obtain high quality Qi to circulate in your body.

4. The Spleen Channel of Foot - Greater Yin (Figure 2-16)
A. Course:
Course #1:

(1). Medial tip of the big toe (Yinbai, Sp-1) - (2). Anterior border of the medial malleolus - (3). Along the posterior border of the tibia - (4). Medial aspect of the leg - (5). Medial aspect of the art. genus - (6). Anterior medial aspect of the thigh - (7). Enter the abdomen - (8). Zhongji (Co-3) and Guanyuan (Co-4)- (9). Pertains to the spleen and communicates with the stomach - (10). Riyue (GB-24) and Qimen (Li-14) - (11). Penetrates the diaphragm through Zhongfu (L-1) - (12). Throat - (13). Root of the tongue.

Course #2:

(9). Stomach - (14). Through the diaphragm and disperses into the heart.

B. Related Viscera:
Spleen (Pertaining Organ), stomach, heart, lung, and intestines.

C. Cavities:
Yinbai (Sp-1), Dadu (Sp-2), Taibai (Sp-3), Gongsun (Sp-4), Shangqiu (Sp-5), Sanyinjiao (Sp-6), Lougu (Sp-7), Diji (Sp-8), Yinlingquan (Sp-9), Xuehai (Sp-10), Jimen (Sp-11), Chongmen (Sp-12), Fushe (Sp-13), Fujie (Sp-14), Daheng (Sp-15), Fuai (Sp-16), Shidou (Sp-17), Tianxi (Sp-18), Xiongxiang (Sp-19), Zhourong (Sp-20), Dabao (Sp-21).

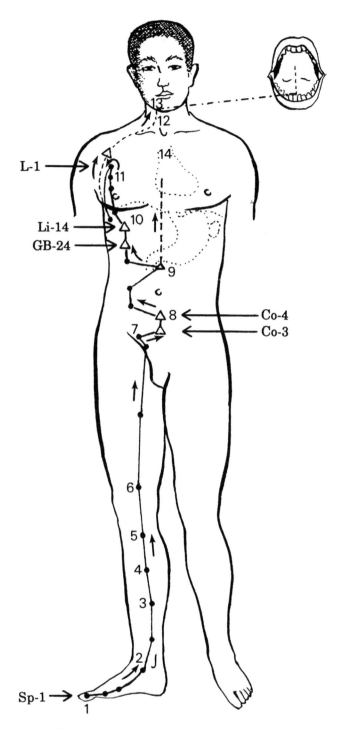

Figure 2-16. The Spleen Channel of the Foot-Greater Yin.

D. Discussion:

The spleen (Yin) and the stomach (Yang) are paired organs. They belong to Earth in the Five Phases, the central direction, the season of long summer (the end of summer), the climatic condition of dampness, the color yellow, the emotion of pensiveness, the taste of sweetness, fragrant odor, and the sound of singing. Their opening is the mouth and they control the flesh and the limbs.

The spleen is the main organ of digestion. Its function is to transport nutrients and regulate the blood (regulate means to keep it within the channels). It is responsible for the transformation of food into nourishment.

When the spleen is weak, the body will not be able to use the nourishment available in food. This will cause general lassitude, fatigue, and a pasty complexion. The upper abdomen is considered the province of the spleen. Deficient spleen Qi is shown by a sense of malaise or fullness in that area. Because it is required that the transportive function of the spleen distribute its Qi upward, weakness in the spleen will usually cause diarrhea. Spleen Qi is also regarded as the Middle Qi, and it is responsible for holding the viscera in place. Insufficiency of the Middle Qi will presage prolapsed stomach, kidneys, etc. In more serious cases, the spleen Yang Qi will be deficient, which is manifested in diarrhea, cold limbs, and abdominal pain that can be soothed by the warmth of frequent hot drinks.

If any of the above symptoms are accompanied by bleeding, especially from the digestive tract or uterus, it is called Spleen Not Controlling the Blood.

Cold and Dampness Harassing the Spleen is a manifestation characterized by a pent-up feeling in the chest and a bloated sensation in the abdomen, lassitude, lack of appetite and taste, a feeling of cold in the limbs, a dark yellowish hue to the skin, some edema and diarrhea or watery stool. The cold and dampness prevent the spleen from performing its transforming and transporting functions. This leads to a great disturbance in water metabolism and is one of the origins of Phlegm.

In Qigong training, one of the final goals is to regulate the Qi flow to its original (normal) level in the five Yin organs. Among them, the spleen is the last and the hardest organ to regulate. It is believed that if you are able to regulate the Qi in your spleen to a normal and healthy level, you will have grasped the key to health and longevity.

5. The Heart Channel of Hand - Lesser Yin (Figure 2-17)
A. Course:
Course #1:
(1). Heart - (2). Lung - (3). Below the axilla - (4). Upper arm - (5). Antecubital fossa - (6). Between ossa metacarpal IV and V - (7). Tip of the little finger (Shaochong, H-9).
Course #2:
(1). Heart - (8). Diaphragm - (9). Small intestine.
Course #3:
(1). Heart - (10). Throat - (11). Tissues surrounding the eye (orbital system).

B. Related Viscera:
Heart (Pertaining Organ), small intestine, lung, and kidney.

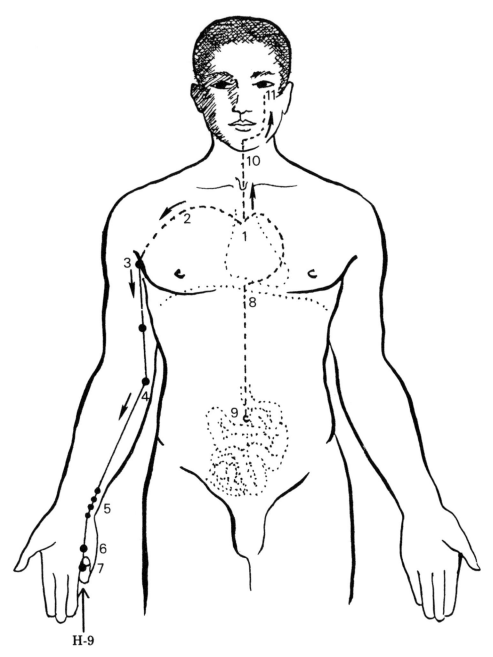

Figure 2-17. The Heart Channel of Hand Lesser Yin.

C. Cavities:

Jiquan (H-1), Qingling (H-2), Shaohai (H-3), Lingdao (H-4), Tongli (H-5), Yinxi (H-6), Shenmen (H-7), Shaofu (H-8), Shaochong (H-9).

D. Discussion:

The heart and the small intestine are paired organs. The heart is considered Yin, and the small intestine is considered Yang, balancing this paired channel. These two organs correspond to Fire in the Five Phases, the southerly direction, the summer season, the climatic condition of heat, the color red, the emotion of happiness, the sound of laughter, the taste of bitterness, and the odor of burning.

Their point of entry is the tongue, they control the blood vessels and are reflected in the face.

Almost all of the problems and disorders of the heart are associated with weakness. The four major types of heart weakness are Deficient Heart Qi, Deficient Heart Yang, Deficient Heart Blood, and Deficient Heart Yin.

The main functions of the heart are associated with the spirit and the blood vessels. The heart governs the blood vessels and is responsible for moving blood through them. It also stores the spirit, and is the organ usually associated with mental processes. Therefore, some forms of emotional distress, dizziness, palpitations, shortness of breath, and lack of vitality are common symptoms of heart ailments. Deficient Heart Qi is symbolized by general lassitude, panting and shallow breathing, and frequent sweating. If the face is swollen and ashen gray or bluish-green, and the limbs are cold, it is called Deficient Heart Yang. The symptoms of restlessness, irritability, dizziness, absentmindedness, and insomnia are typical signs of Deficient Heart Blood. In Deficient Heart Yin cases, developments with a flushed feeling in the palms and face, low grade fever, and night sweating will occur.

The symptom of Heart Excess arises from an excess of Heart Fire. This is manifested by fever, occasionally accompanied by delirium, a racking pulse, intense restlessness, insomnia or frequent nightmares, a bright red face, a red or blistered and painful tongue, and often a burning sensation during urination. The latter symptom is the result of Heat being transferred from the heart to the small intestine, which interferes with the small intestine's role in metabolism and the body's management of water.

In Qigong society, it is believed that the mind is associated with the heart, and that it is also directly related to the spirit. The term heart (Xin) is usually used to represent the emotional mind or ideas. The Middle Dan Tian at the solar plexus is considered the residence of the Fire Qi. This Fire is used to nourish the brain and the spirit (Shen) at its residence, the Upper Dan Tian or third eye. In Chinese medicine it is said that the heart is the temple of the spirit because it supplies Fire Qi and can nourish the spirit without limit.

Generally speaking, the heart is very sensitive during the summertime. The heart is a Yin channel, and when the summer Yang comes it can increase the heart's Qi level and cause problems. Emotional disturbances, such as excitement from happiness, are considered harmful to the heart as well, especially during the summertime. Qigong emphasizes regulating the heart in the summer.

6. The Small Intestine Channel of Hand - Greater Yang
(Figure 2-18)

A. Course:

Course #1:

(1). Tip of the digitus minimus (Shaoze, SI-1) - (2). Wrist - (3). Top of the elbow - (4). Dorsal surface of the upper arm - (5). Shoulder -

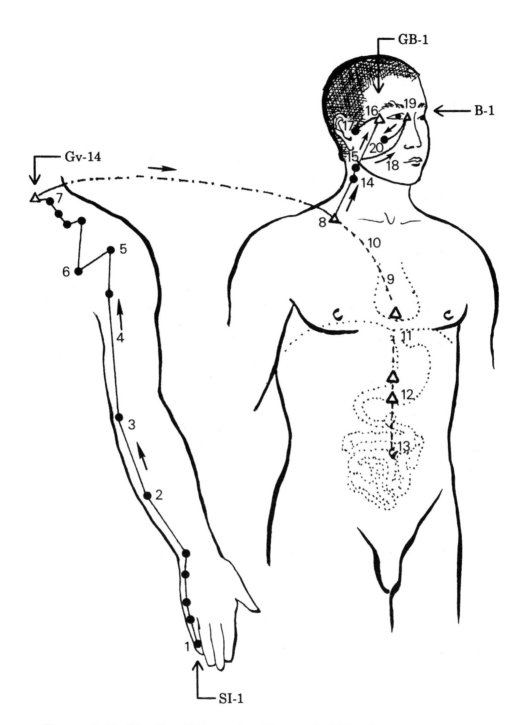

Figure 2-18. The Small Intestine Channel of Hand-Greater Yang.

(6). Circle around the superior and inferior fossa of the scapula - (7).
Meets Dazhui (Gv-14) - (8). Enters the supraclavicular fossa - (9).
Heart - (10). Passes along the esophagus - (11). Diaphragm - (12).
Stomach - (13). Small intestine.

    Course #2:

    (8). Supraclavicular fossa - (14). Neck - (15). Cheek - (16).
Tongziliao (GB-1) - (17). Into the ear.

Course #3:

(18). Cheek - (19). Jingming (B-1) - (20). Distributes over zygoma obliquely.

B. Related Viscera:

Small intestine (Pertaining Organ), heart, and stomach.

C. Cavities:

Shaoze (SI-1), Qiangu (SI-2), Houxi (SI-3), Hand-Wangu (SI-4), Yanggu (SI-5), Yanglao (SI-6), Zhizheng (SI-7), Xiaohai (SI-8), Jianzhen (SI-9), Naoshu (SI-10), Tianzong (SI-11), Bingfeng (SI-12), Quyuan (SI-13), Jianwaishu (SI-14), Jianzhongshu (SI-15), Tianchuang (SI-16), Tianrong (SI-17), Quanliao (SI-18), Tinggong (SI-19).

D. Discussion:

The heart and the small intestine are paired organs. The heart is considered Yin, and the small intestine is considered Yang, balancing this paired channel. These two organs correspond to Fire in the Five Phases, the southerly direction, the summer season, the climatic condition of heat, the color red, the emotion of happiness, the sound of laughter, the taste of bitterness, and the odor of burning. Their point of entry is the tongue. They control the blood vessels and are reflected in the face.

The major function of the small intestine is to separate waste material from the nutritious elements in food. The nutritious elements are then distributed throughout the body and the waste is sent on to the large intestine.

The small and large intestines are located in the Lower Dan Tian. In order to store the Original Qi converted from Original Essence, the abdomen must be healthy and the Qi circulation in the area of the intestines must be smooth and natural. The best way to reach this goal is through abdominal breathing exercises. One such exercise is to lead the Original Qi upward following the heart and small intestine Qi channels to cool down the heart Fire.

7. The Urinary Bladder Channel of Foot - Greater Yang
(Figure 2-19)

A. Course:

Course #1:

(1). Canthus medial - (2). Shenting (Gv-24) - (3). Baihui (Gv-20).

Course #2:

(3). Baihui (Gv-20) - (4). Fubai (GB-10), Head-Qiaoyin (GB-11), and Wangu (Head-Wangu, GB-12), etc.

Course #3:

(3). Baihui (Gv-20) - (5). Naohu (Gv-17) - (6). Neck - (7). Dazhui (Gv-14) and Taodao (Gv-13) - (8). Lumber region - (9). Kidney - (10). Urinary bladder.

Course #4:

(8). Lumbar region - (11). Crosses the buttock - (12). Popliteal fossa.

Course #5:

Figure 2-19. The Urinary Bladder Channel of Foot-Greater Yang.

(6). Neck - (13). Medial side of the scapula - (14). Lumber region - (15). Lateral side of the thigh - (16). Popliteal fossa - (17). M. gastrocnemius - (18). Pushen (B-61)- (19). The lateral side of the tip of the small toe (Zhiyin, B-67).

B. Related Viscera:

Urinary bladder (Pertaining Organ), kidney, brain, and heart.

C. Cavities:

Jingming (B-1), Zanzhu (B-2), Meichong (B-3), Quchai (B-4), Wuchu (B-5), Chengguang (B-6), Tongtian (B-7), Luogue (B-8), Yuzhen (B-9), Tianzhu (B-10), Dashu (B-11), Fengmen (B-12), Feishu (B-13), Jueyinshu (B-14), Xinshu (B-15), Dushu (B-16), Geshu (B-17), Ganshu (B-18), Danshu (B-19), Pishu (B-20), Weishu (B-21), Sanjiaoshu (B-22), Shenshu (B-23), Qihaishu (B-24), Dachangshu (B-25), Guanyuanshu (B-26), Xiaochangshu (B-27), Pangguanshu (B-28), Zhonglushu (B-29), Baihuanshu (B-30), Shangliao (B-31), Ciliao (B-32), Zhongliao (B-33), Xialiao (B-34), Huiyang (B-35), Fufen (B-36), Pohu (B-37), Gaohuangshu (B-38), Shentang (B-39), Yixi (B-40), Geguan (B-41), Hunmen (B-42), Yanggang (B-43), Yishe (B-44), Weicang (B-45), Huangmen (B-46), Zhishi (B-47), Baohuang (B-48), Zhibian (B-49), Chengfu (B-50), Yinmen (B-51), Fuxi (B-52), Weiyang (B-53), Weizhong (B-54), Heyang (B-55), Chengjin (B-56), Chengshan (B-57), Feiyang (B-58), Fuyang (B-59), Kunlun (B-60), Pushen (B-61), Shenmai (B-62), Jinmen (B-63), Jinggu (B-64), Shugu (B-65), Foot-Tonggu (B-66), and Zhiyin (B-67).

D. Discussion:

The kidneys (Yin) and the urinary bladder (Yang) are paired organs. They correspond to Water in the Five Phases, the winter season, the cold climatic condition, the southerly direction, the color black, the emotion of fear, the taste of salt, the smell of decay, and the sound of groaning. Their sensory organ is the ear. Their opening is the urethra. They control the bones, marrow, and brain, and their health is reflected in the hair of the head.

The main function of the urinary bladder is to transform fluids into urine and excrete it from the body.

In Qigong, the urinary bladder has never enjoyed serious attention. However, its pairing partner the kidney is one of the most important organs - one with which all Qigong practitioners are concerned and train most often. The reason for this is simply that the kidneys are the residence of the Original Essence.

8. The Kidney Channel of Foot - Lesser Yin (Figure 2-20)

A. Course:

Course #1:

(1). Small toe - (2). Inferior aspect of the navicular tuberosity (Rangu, K-2) - (3). Behind the malleolus medialis - (4). Spreads to the heel - (5). M. gastrocnemius - (6). Medial side of the popliteal fossa - (7). Posterior aspect of the thigh - (8). Enters kidney - (9). Communicates with the urinary bladder - (10). Guanyuan (Co-4) and Zhongji (Co-3).

Course #2:

(9). Kidney - (11). Liver and diaphragm - (12). Enters the lung - (13). Along the throat - (14). Root of the tongue.

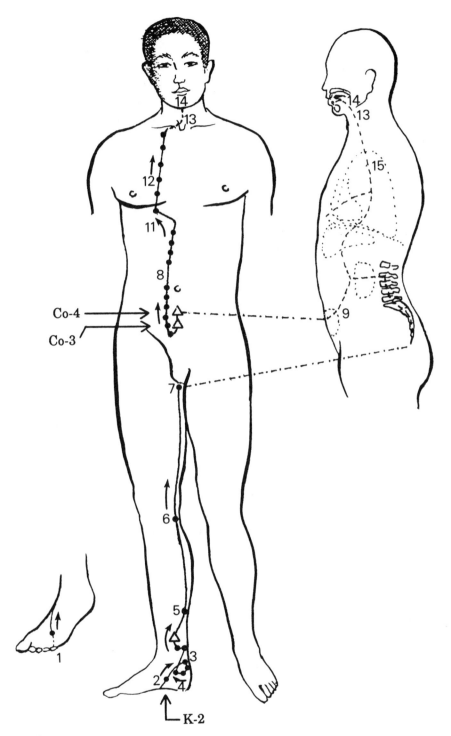

Figure 2-20. The Kidney Channel of Foot-Lesser Yang.

Course #3:
(12). Lung - (15). Heart and spreads to the chest.

B. Related Viscera:

Kidney (Pertaining Organ), urinary bladder, liver, lung, heart, and other organs.

C. Cavities:

Yongquan (K-1), Rangu (K-2), Taixi (K-3), Dazhong (K-4), Shuiquan (K-5), Zhaohai (K-6), Fuliu (K-7), Jiaoxin (K-8), Zhubin (K-9), Yingu (K-10), Henggu (K-11), Dahe (K-12), Qixue (K-13), Siman (K-14), Abdomen-Zhongzhu (K-15), Huangshu (K-16), Shangqu (K-17), Shiguan (K-18), Yindu (K-19), Abdomen-Tonggu (K-20), Youmen (K-21), Bulang (K-22), Shenfeng (K-23), Lingxu (K-24), Shencang (K-25), Yuzhong (K-26), and Shufu (K-27).

D. Discussion:

The kidneys (Yin) and the urinary bladder (Yang) are paired organs. They correspond to Water in the Five Phases, the winter season, the cold climatic condition, the southerly direction, the color black, the emotion of fear, the taste of salt, a rotten smell, and the sound of groaning. Their sensory organ is the ear. Their opening is the urethra. They control the bones, marrow, and brain, and their health is reflected in the hair of the head.

The kidneys store Original Essence (Yuan Jing) and are therefore responsible for growth, development, and reproductive functions. They play the primary role in water metabolism and control the body's liquids, and also hold the body's most fundamental Yin and Yang.

Because the kidneys are the repositories of the basal Yin and Yang of the body, any disorder, if sufficiently chronic, will involve the kidneys. More significantly, a disease of the kidneys will usually lead to problems in other organs. Methods of strengthening the kidneys are therefore used by both medical and Qigong societies to increase or maintain vitality and health. The symptoms of Deficient Kidney Yang or Yin are typical symptoms of the disorder, and will appear to a certain extent as Deficient Yang or Yin patterns in any organ.

It is easy to understand and memorize the symptoms of Deficient Kidney Yin if one learns the correspondences of the kidneys and remembers that Yin represents the constructive, nourishing, and fluid aspects of the body. Usually, the lower back is weak and sore, there is ringing in the ears and loss of hearing acuity, the face is ashen or dark, especially under the eyes. It is common to feel dizziness and thirst, and to experience night sweats and low grade fevers. In addition, men have little semen and tend toward premature ejaculation, while women have little or no menstruation.

Deficient Kidney Yang symptoms are significantly associated with loss of energy or warmth. Similar to Deficient Kidney Yin, there is commonly ringing in the ears, dizziness, and soreness in the lower back. However, the soreness is characterized by a feeling of coldness, lassitude, and fatigue. Weakness in the legs can be noticed. In men, there is a tendency toward impotence, and in both sexes, clear and voluminous urine or incontinence.

Usually, Deficient Kidney Yin generates similar disorders in the heart and liver, while Deficient Kidney Yang disturbs the functions of the spleen and lungs. The progression could be in the opposite direction. When this pattern is associated with the lungs, it is called

"Kidney Not Receiving Qi," a type of wheezing characterized by difficult breathing, mainly during inhalation. In addition to the Deficient Kidney Yang symptoms, this condition is also manifested by a faint voice, coughing, puffiness in the face, and spontaneous sweating.

The kidneys perform an important role in the metabolism of water. If these functions are disrupted, the condition of Deficient Kidneys will lead to Spreading Water.

In Qigong practice, essence (Jing) is considered the most original source of human vitality. Qi is converted from essence, and this Qi supplies the entire body and nourishes the brain and spirit. It is believed by both Chinese medical and Qigong societies that the kidneys are the residence of Original Essence. In order to protect your inherent essence, you must strengthen your kidneys. Only when your kidneys are strong will you be able to keep your essence at its residence. Therefore, keeping the kidneys healthy has become one of the most important subjects in Qigong.

Maintaining the kidneys in a healthy state includes protecting the physical kidneys from degeneration, and maintaining a smooth and correct level of Qi flow. In order to reach this goal, the diet must be considered. For example, too much salt is harmful to the kidneys, and eating too much eggplant will weaken the kidneys. In addition, the condition of the body is also important. Such things as overworking without proper rest will increase tension on the kidneys and make the Qi flow stagnant. In winter, the kidneys will have more tension than in summer. Due to this, the Qi flow is more stagnant in the wintertime than in the summertime. Consequently, back pain problems increase in the winter.

In order to protect the kidneys, Qigong practitioners have studied the relationship of the kidneys to nature, food, and even to emotional states. They have developed massage techniques and specific exercises to increase Qi circulation in the kidneys during the winter. Since the health of the kidneys is related to the emotions as well, learning how to regulate the mind in order to regulate the Qi has become one of the major training goals in Qigong.

9. The Pericardium Channel of Hand - Absolute Yin (Figure 2-21)

A. Course:

Course #1:

(1). Pericardium - (2). Below the armpit - (3). Axilla - (4). Forearm - (5). Wrist - (6). Palm - (7). Tip of middle finger (Zhongchong, P-9).

Course #2:

(1). Pericardium - (8). Diaphragm - (9). Connects triple burner (Sanjiao)

Course #3:

(6). Palm (Laogong, P-8) - (10). Tip of ring finger (Guanchong, TB-1).

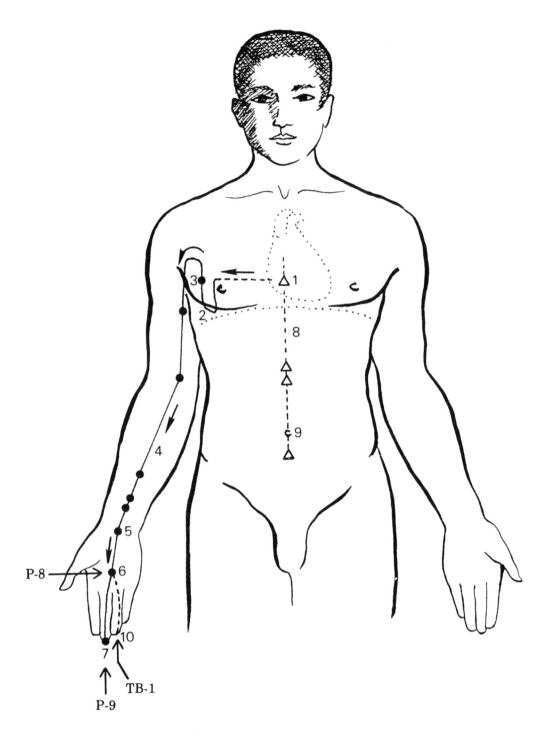

Figure 2-21. The Pericardium Channel of Hand-Absolute Yin.

B. Related Viscera:

Pericardium (Pertaining Organ) and triple burner (Sanjiao).

C. Cavities:

Tianchi (P-1), Tianquan (P-2), Quze (P-3), Ximen (P-4), Jianshi (P-5), Neiguan (P-6), Daling (P-7), Laogong (P-8), and Zhongchong (P-9).

D. Discussion:

The pericardium (Yin) and the triple burner (Yang) are paired organs. They are said to correspond to the "Ministerial Fire," as opposed to the "Sovereign Fire" of the heart and small intestine. Though the pericardium has no separate physiological functions, it is generally mentioned with regard to the delirium induced by high fevers.

The regulation of Qi in the pericardium is considered a very important subject in Qigong. It is believed that the heart, the most vital organ in your body, must have a proper level of Qi circulation in order to function normally. The Qi level of the heart can be raised easily to an abnormal state by illness, emotional disturbance, exercise, or injury. The function of the pericardium is to dissipate the excess Qi from the heart and direct it to the Laogong cavity (P-8), located in the center of the palm. From Laogong, the excess Qi will be released naturally and hence, regulate the heart's Qi level. The Laogong cavity is used in Qigong massage to reduce the body's temperature during a fever. You can see that the purpose of the pericardium is to regulate the Qi in the heart through the Laogong cavity.

You should understand that in Qigong it is believed that there are five centers (called gates) where the Qi of the body is able to communicate with the surrounding environment, and, consequently, regulate the Qi level in your body. Two of these five centers are the Laogong cavities, and two others are the Yongquan cavities (K-1), used to regulate the Qi in the kidneys. The fifth one is your face. The face is connected and related to many of your organs. Whenever any of your organ Qi is not normal, it shows on your face.

10. The Triple Burner Channel of Hand - Lesser Yang (Figure 2-22)

A. Course:

Course #1:

(1). Tip of the ring finger (Guanchong, TB-1) - (2). Between the ossa metacarpal IV and V - (3). Wrist - (4). Dorsal side of the forearm - (5). Passing the olecranon - (6). Lateral aspect of the upper arm - (7). Shoulder - (8). Jianjing (GB-21) - (9). Enters the supraclavicular fossa - (10). Branches out in the chest, communicating with the pericardium - (11). Diaphragm - (12). Links successively the upper, middle, and lower portions of the body cavity.

Course #2:

(10). Shanzhong (Co-17) - (13). Supraclavicular fossa - (14). Neck - (15). Dazhui (Gv-14) - (16). Posterior border of the ear - (17). Xuanli (GB-6) and Hanyan (GB-4) - (18). Quanliao (SI-18).

Course #3:

(19). Retro-auricular region where it enters the ear - (20). Emerges in front of the ear - (21). Lateral canthus.

B. Related Viscera:

It pertains to the upper, middle and lower portions of the body cavity (Sanjiao) and communicates with the pericardium.

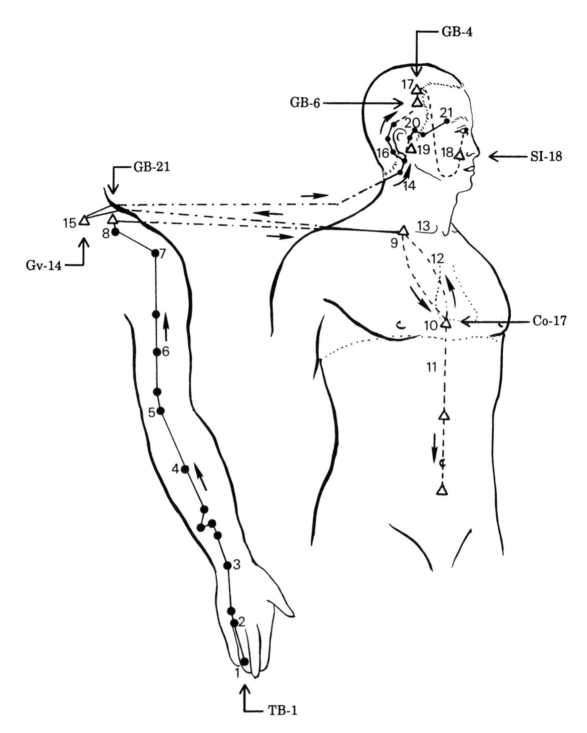

Figure 2-22. The Triple Burner Channel of Hand-Lesser Yang.

C. Cavities:

Guanchong (TB-1), Yemen (TB-2), Hand-Zhongzhu (TB-3), Yangchi (TB-4), Waiguan (TB-5), Zhigou (TB-6), Huizong (TB-7), Sanyangluo (TB-8), Sidu (TB-9), Tianjing (TB-10), Qinglengyuan (TB-11), Xiaoluo (TB-12), Naohui (TB-13), Jianliao (TB-14), Tianliao (TB-15), Tianyou (TB-16), Yifeng (TB-17), Qimai (TB-18), Luxi (TB-

19), Jiaosun (TB-20), Ermen (TB-21), Ear-Heliao (TB-22), and Sizhukong (TB-23).

D. Discussion:

At least as far back as the 3rd century A.D., in the "Classic of Difficulties" (Nan Jing) the triple burner was regarded as "having a name but no form." In the "Inner Classic" (Nei Jing), the triple burner was considered an organ that coordinated all the functions of water metabolism. In other traditional documents, the burners were considered three regions of the body that were used to group the organs. The upper burner includes the chest, neck, and head as well as the functions of the heart and lungs. The middle burner is the region between the chest and the navel, and includes the functions of the stomach, liver, and spleen. The lower burner spans the lower abdomen, and the functions of the kidneys and urinary bladder. Therefore, the upper burner has been compared to a mist which spreads the blood and Qi, the middle burner is like a foam which churns up food in the process of digestion, and the lower burner resembles a swamp where all the impure substances are excreted.

Regulating the Qi to a normally "smooth-flow" state is one of the main Qigong training methods for maintaining health. It is normally done through Wai Dan exercises, and it is believed that the Qi must flow around internal organs smoothly in order for them to maintain their normal functions. This means that in order to keep Qi flow smooth and the organs healthy, you must first learn how to regulate and relax muscles that are holding and related to a given organ. External movements also exercise internal muscles. One of the most common external exercises is regulating the triple burner by lifting your hands up above your head and then moving them down slowly. These up and down arm movements extend and relax the internal muscles and thereby increase Qi flow.

11. The Gall Bladder Channel of Foot - Lesser Yang (Figure 2-23)
A. Course:

Course #1:

(1). Outer canthus of the eye (Tongziliao, GB-1) - (2). Nose-Heliao (TB-22) - (3). Jiaosun (TB-20) - (4). Dazhui (Gv-14) - (5). Enters the supraclavicular fossa.

Course #2:

(6). Retro-auricular region, passes through Yifeng (TB-17) - (7). Tinggong (SI-19) and Xiaguan (S-7).

Course #3:

(1). Outer canthus of the eye - (8). Daying (S-5) - (9). Infraorbital region - (10). Jiache (S-6) - (11). Supraclavicular fossa - (12). Into the chest - (13). Tianchi (P-1) - (14). Communicates with the liver - (15). Pertains to the gall bladder - (16). Inside of the hypochondrium - (17). Around the genitals - (18). Hip (Huantiao, GB-30).

Course #4:

(19). Supraclavicular fossa - (20). Axilla - (21). Lateral aspect of the chest - (22). Through the hypochondrium - (23). Zhangmen (Li-

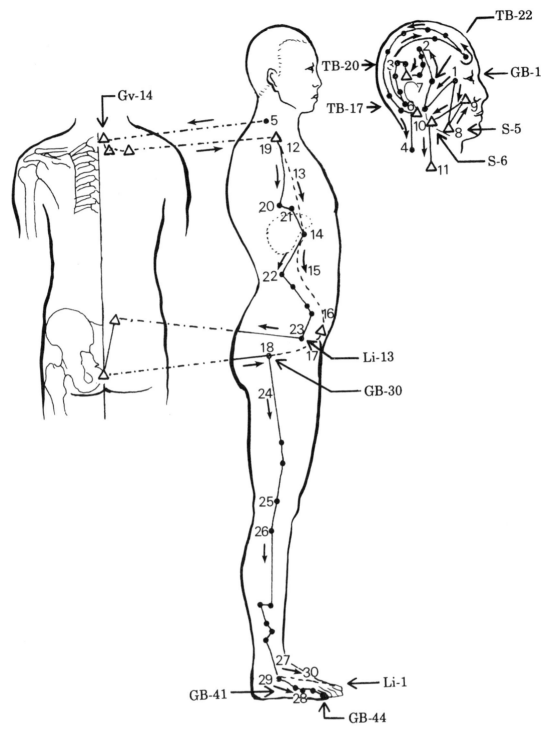

Figure 2-23. The Gall Bladder Channel of Foot-Lesser Yang.

13) - (24). Along the lateral aspect of thigh - (25). Knee - (26).
Anterior aspect of the fibula - (27). Anterior aspect of the malleolus -
(28). Lateral side of the tip of the 4th toe or Zuqiaoyin (GB-44).
  Course #5:
  (29). Dorsum of the foot (Linqi, GB-41) - (30). Big toe (Dadun, Li-1).

B. Related Viscera:
Gall bladder (Pertaining Organ), liver, and heart.

C. Cavities:
Tongziliao (GB-1), Tinghui (GB-2), Shangguan (GB-3), Hanyan (GB-4), Xuanlu (GB-5), Xuanli (GB-6), Qubin (GB-7), Shuaigu (GB-8), Tianchong (GB-9), Fubai (GB-10), Head-Qiaoyin (GB-11), Head-Wangu (GB-12), Benshen (GB-13), Yangbai (GB-14), Head-Linqi (GB-15), Muchuang (GB-16), Zhengying (GB-17), Chengling (GB-18), Naokong (GB-19), Fengchi (GB-20), Jianjing (GB-21), Yuanye (GB-22), Zhejin (GB-23), Riyue (GB-24), Jingmen (GB-25), Daimai (GB-26), Wushu (GB-27), Weidao (GB-28), Femur-Juliao (GB-29), Huantiao (GB-30), Fengshi (GB-31), Femur-Zhongdu (GB-32), Xiyangguan (GB-33), Yanglingquan (GB-34), Yangjiao (GB-35), Waiqiu (GB-36), Guangming (GB-37), Yangfu (GB-38), Xuanzhong (GB-39), Qiuxu (GB-40), Foot-Linqi (GB-41), Diwuhui (GB-42), Xiaxi (GB-43), Foot-Qiaoyin (GB-44).

D. Discussion:
The liver (Yin) and the gall bladder (Yang) are paired organs. They correspond to Wood in the Five Phases, the direction east, the spring season, the climatic wind, the color green, the emotion of anger, the taste of sourness, the goatish odor, and the sound of shouting. Their point of entry is the eyes. They control the sinews (muscles and joints), and their health is reflected in the finger and toe nails.

The main function of the gall bladder is storing and excreting the bile produced by the liver. Together with the heart, the gall bladder is responsible for decision-making.

The main disease related to the gall bladder is a disorder affecting the flow of bile, usually caused by Dampness and Heat. This is commonly manifested by pain in the region of the liver, an oppressive sensation of fullness in the abdomen, and yellowish eyes, skin, urine, and tongue.

The gall bladder has never enjoyed serious attention during Qigong training. Its paired partner the liver however, has received much more attention.

12. The Liver Channel of Foot - Absolute Yin (Figure 2-24)
A. Course:
Course #1:

(1). Behind the nail of the big toe - (2). Malleolus medialis - (3). Sanyinjiao (Sp-6) - (4). Side of shin - (5). Side of knee - (6). Medial aspect of the thigh - (7). Chongmen (Sp-12) and Fushe (Sp-13) - (8). Pubic region - (9). Lower abdomen - (10). Qugu (Co-2), Zhongli (Co-3), and Guanyuan (Co-4) - (11). Liver - (12). Lower chest - (13). Neck posterior - (14). Upper palate - (15). Tissues of the eye - (16). Forehead - (17). Vertex.

Course #2:

(15). Eye - (18). Cheek - (19). Curves around the inner surface of the lips.

Figure 2-24. The Liver Channel of Foot-Absolute Yin.

Course #3:
(20). Liver - (21). Through diaphragm - (22). Lung.

B. Related Viscera:

Liver (Pertaining Organ), gall bladder, lung, stomach, and brain.

C. Cavities:

Dadun (L-1), Xingjian (L-2), Taichong (L-3), Zhongfeng (L-4), Ligou (L-5), Tibia-Zhongdu (L-6), Xiguan (L-7), Ququan (L-8), Yinbao

(L-9), Femur-Wuli (L-10), Yinlian (L-11), Jimai (L-12), Zhangmen (L-13), and Qimen (L-14).

D. Discussion:

The liver (Yin) and the gall bladder (Yang) are considered paired organs. They correspond to Wood in the Five Phases, the direction east, the spring season, the climatic condition of wind, the color green, the emotion of anger, the taste of sourness, the goatish odor, and the sound of shouting. Their point of entry is the eyes. They control the sinews (muscles and joints), and their health is reflected in the finger and toe nails.

The main task of the liver is spreading and regulating Qi throughout the entire body. Its unique character is flowing and free. Therefore, depression or frustration can disturb the functioning of the liver. In addition, the liver is also responsible for storing blood when the body is at rest. This characteristic, together with its control over the lower abdomen, makes it the most critical organ in regards to women's menstrual cycle and sexuality.

Depression or long-term frustration can stagnate the liver's spreading function and result in continuing depression, a bad temper, and a painful, swollen feeling in the chest and sides. If this condition worsens, it may cause disharmony between the liver and the stomach and/or spleen. This disorder is symbolized by the "rebellion" of Qi in the latter organs, whereby Qi moves in the opposite direction than is normal. For example, the stomach Qi normally descends, so rebellious Qi means hiccoughing, vomiting, etc. In the case of the spleen, the Qi ordinarily moves upward, so rebellious Qi in this organ means diarrhea.

Depression of the liver Qi is the main cause of many women's disorders, including menstrual irregularities, swollen and painful breasts, etc.

One of the most important responsibilities of the liver is the storage of blood with intended emphasis upon nourishing and moistening. Whenever the liver blood is deficient, the liver will not be able to handle the function of moistening. This is generally shown as dry and painful eyes with blurred or weak vision, lack of suppleness or pain in moving the joints, dry skin, dizziness, and infrequent or spotty menstruation. If the Deficient Liver Yin has become serious, the conditions Rising Liver Fire or Hyper Liver Yang Ascending occur. These occurrences are evidenced in ill-temper, restlessness, headache, vertigo, red face and eyes, and a parched mouth. If the liver Yin is so deficient that it is incapable of securing the liver Yang, many of the symptoms appear as disorders of the head. Weakness in the lower joints may also be manifested.

The liver is one of the five Yin organs whose Qi level the Qigong practitioner wants to regulate. Since the liver and the gall bladder are directly connected, when the liver's Qi is regulated, the Qi circulating in the gall bladder will also be regulated. Many methods have been developed for regulating the liver Qi. Wai Dan Qigong works through the limbs. For example, when the arms are moved up and down, the internal muscles surrounding the liver will be moved and the Qi around the liver will be circulated smoothly. In Nei Dan Qigong, it is believed that the liver is closely related to your mind. It is also believed that when your mind is regulated, the Qi circulation in the liver will be normal and therefore the liver will function properly.

Important Points

1. The spleen, liver, and heart are the organs with the most direct relationship with the blood. The spleen filters the blood (modifying the blood's structure), the liver stores the blood, and the heart moves it. Any problem associated with the blood will involve at least one of these organs.

2. The liver and the kidney are closely related. Their channels cross in many places. The liver stores blood; the kidney stores essence. These substances, both of which are Yin, have a considerable influence on the reproductive functions.

3. The heart (upper burner, Fire) and the kidney (lower burner, Water) keep each other in check and are dependent upon one another. The spirit of the heart and the essence of the kidneys cooperate in establishing and maintaining human consciousness.

4. The spleen's digestive function is associated with the distributive functions of the liver. Disharmony between these two results in various digestive troubles. The transportive and digestive functions of the spleen (also called the Middle Qi) depend upon the strength of the kidney Yang.

5. Although the lungs govern Qi, Qi from the lungs must mix with essence from the kidneys before Original Qi can be produced. The lungs govern Qi, the liver spreads Qi, and the kidneys provide its basis.

The Eight Extraordinary Qi Vessels

The eight extraordinary Qi vessels and the twelve primary Qi channels (meridians) comprise the main part of the channel system. Most of the eight vessels branch out from the twelve primary channels and share the function of circulating Qi throughout the body. These vessels form a web of complex interconnections with the channels. At the same time, each has its own functional characteristics and clinical utility independent of the channels.

Traditional Chinese medicine emphasizes the twelve primary organ-related channels and only two of the eight vessels (the Governing and the Conception vessels). The other six vessels are not used very often simply because they are not understood as well as the other channels, and there is still a lot of research being conducted on them. Although they were discovered two thousand years ago, little has been written about them. There is a lot of research on the extraordinary vessels being conducted today, especially in Japan, but the results of one researcher often contradict the results that another has achieved.

In this subsection we would like to compile and summarize the important points from the limited number of available documents. Since references from original Chinese sources are very scarce, and references from Western textbooks are tentative, esoteric, or in disagreement with one another, I have used my own judgement in selecting ideas and details. Before reviewing these eight vessels, we will first define them and then summarize their functions.

What are the Eight Vessels?

The eight vessels are called "Qi Jing Ba Mai." Qi means odd, strange, or mysterious. Jing means meridian or channels. Ba means eight and Mai means vessels. Qi Jing Ba Mai is then translated as "Odd Meridians and Eight Vessels" or "Extraordinary Meridians (EM)." "Odd" has a meaning of strange in Chinese. It is used simply because these eight vessels are not well understood yet. Many Chinese doctors explain that they are called "Odd" simply because there are four vessels that are not paired. Since these eight vessels also contribute to the maintenance of homeostasis, sometimes they are called "Homeostatic Meridians." French acupuncturists call them "Miraculous Meridians" because they were able to create therapeutic effects when all other techniques had failed. In addition, because each of these channels exerts a strong effect upon psychic functioning and individuality, t he command points are among the most important psychological points in the body. For this reason, they are occasionally called "The Eight Psychic Channels."

These vessels are: 1. Governing Vessel (Du Mai); 2. Conception Vessel (Ren Mai); 3. Thrusting Vessel (Chong Mai); 4. Girdle Vessel (Dai Mai); 5. Yang Heel Vessel (Yangqiao Mai); 6. Yin Heel Vessel (Yinqiao Mai); 7. Yang Linking Vessel (Yangwei Mai); and 8. Yin Linking Vessel (Yinwei Mai).

General Functions of the Eight Vessels

1. Serve as Qi Reservoirs:

Because the eight vessels are so different from each other, it is difficult to generalize their characteristics and functions. However, one of the most common characteristics of the eight vessels was specified by Bian Que in his "Nan Jing." He reported that **THE TWELVE ORGAN-RELATED QI CHANNELS CONSTITUTE RIVERS, AND THE EIGHT EXTRAORDINARY VESSELS CONSTITUTE RESERVOIRS**. These reservoirs, especially the Conception and Governing vessels, absorb excess Qi from the main channels, and then return it when they are deficient.

You should understand however, that because of the limited number of traditional documents, as well as the lack of modern, scientific methods of Qi research, it is difficult to determine the precise behavior and characteristics of these eight vessels. They can be understood on a number of different levels, and they perform different functions and contain every kind of Qi such as Ying Qi, Wei Qi, Jing Qi, and even blood.

When the twelve primary channels are deficient in Qi, the eight vessels will supply it. This store of Qi can easily be tapped into with acupuncture needles through those cavities connecting the eight vessels to the twelve channels. The connection cavities behave like the gates of a reservoir, which can be used to adjust the strength of the Qi flow in the rivers and the level of Qi in the reservoir. Sometimes, when it is necessary, the reservoir will release Qi by itself. For example, when a person has had a shock, either physically or mentally, the Qi in some of the main channels will be deficient. This will cause particular organs to be stressed, and Qi will accumulate rapidly around these organs. When this happens, the reservoir must release Qi to increase the deficient circulation and prevent further damage.

2. Guard Specific Areas Against 'Evil Qi':

The Qi which protects the body from outside intruders is called "Wei Qi" (Guardian Qi). Among the eight vessels, the Thrusting vessel, the Governing vessel, and the Conception vessel play major roles in guarding the abdomen, thorax, and the back.

3. Regulate the Changes of Life Cycles:

According to Chapter 1 of "Su Wen," the Thrusting vessel and the Conception vessel also regulate the changes of the life cycles which occur at 7 year intervals for women and 8 year intervals for men.

4. Circulate Jing Qi to the Entire Body, Particularly the Five 'Ancestral Organs':

One of the most important functions of the eight vessels is to deliver Jing Qi (Essence Qi, which has been converted from Original Essence and sexual essence) to the entire body, including the skin and hair. They must also deliver Jing Qi to the five ancestral organs: the brain and spinal cord, the liver and gall bladder, the bone marrow, the uterus, and the blood system.

1. The Governing Vessel (Du Mai) (Figure 2-25)
A. Course:
Course #1:

(1). Perineum - (2). Along the middle of the spine - (3). Fengfu (Gv-16) - (4). Enters the brain - (5). To the top of the head - (6). Midline of the forehead across the bridge of the nose - (7). Upper lip.

Course #2:

(8). Pelvic region - (9). Descends to the genitals and perineum - (10). Tip of the coccyx - (11). Gluteal region (intersects the kidney and urinary bladder channels) - (12). Returns to the spinal column and then joins with the kidneys.

Course #3:

(13). Inner canthus of the eye - (14). Two (bilateral) branches, ascend across the forehead - (15). Converge at the vertex (enters the brain) - (16). Emerges at the lower end of the nape of the neck - (17).

Figure 2-25. The Governing Vessel (Du Mai).

Divides into two branches which descend along opposite sides of the spine to the waist - (18). Kidneys.

Course #4.

(19). Lower abdomen - (20). Across the navel - (21). Passes through the heart - (22). Enters the trachea - (23). Crosses the cheek and encircles the mouth - (24). Terminates at a point below the middle of the eye.

***This vessel intersects Fengmen (B-12) and Huiyin (Co-1).

B. Cavities:

Changqiang (Gv-1), Yaoshu (Gv-2), Yaoyanggguan (Gv-3), Mingmen (Gv-4), Xuanshu (Gv-5), Jizhong (Gv-6), Zhongshu (Gv-7), Jinsuo (Gv-8), Zhiyang (Gv-9), Lingtai (Gv-10), Shendao (Gv-11), Shenzhu (Gv-12), Taodao (Gv-13), Dazhui (Gv-14), Yamen (Gv-15), Fengfu (Gv-16), Naohu (Gv-17), Qiangjian (Gv-18), Houding (Gv-19), Baihui (Gv-20), Qianding (Gv-21), Xinhui (Gv-22), Shangxing (Gv-23), Shenting (Gv-24), Suliao (Gv-25), Renzhong (Gv-26), Duiduan (Gv-27), and Yinjiao (Gv-28).

C. Discussion:

The Governing Vessel is the confluence of all the Yang channels, over which it is said to "govern." Because it controls all the Yang channels, it is called the "Sea of Yang Meridians." This is apparent from its pathway because it flows up the midline of the back, a Yang area, and in the center of all Yang channels (except the stomach channel which flows in the front). The Governing Vessel governs all the Yang channels, which means that it can be used to increase the Yang energy of the body.

Since the Governing Vessel is the "Sea of Yang Meridians" and it controls or governs the back, the area richest in Guardian Qi (Wei Qi), it is also responsible for the circulation of the body's Guardian Qi to guard against external evil intruders. The circulation of Guardian Qi starts from Fengfu (Gv-16), and moves down the Governing Vessel to Huiyin (Co-1). It is said that it takes 21 days for the Guardian Qi to flow from Fengfu to Huiyin, and 9 days from Huiyin to the throat, making it a monthly cycle.

According to Chinese medical science, Guardian Qi is Yang Qi and therefore represents the "Fire" of the body. Its quick and ubiquitous circulation keeps the fire going in the body and controls the loss of body heat. Guardian Qi is also inextricably linked with the fluids that flow outside the channels, in the skin and flesh. Consequently, through the breathing (under control of the lungs), Guardian Qi is responsible for the opening and the closing of the pores, and also controls sweating.

The Governing vessel is also responsible for nourishing the five ancestral organs, which include the brain and spinal cord. This is one of the ways in which the kidneys "control" the brain, as is said in Chinese medicine.

Because of their importance to health, the Governing vessel and the Conception vessel are considered the two most important Qi channels to be trained in Qigong, especially in Nei Dan. Training related to these two vessels includes: 1. How to fill them with Qi so that you have enough to regulate the twelve channels, 2. How to open up stagnant areas in these two vessels so that the Qi flows smoothly and strongly, 3. How to effectively direct the Qi to nourish the brain and raise up the Shen, 4. How to effectively govern the Qi in the twelve channels, and nourish the organs, 5. How to use your raised Shen to lead the Guardian Qi to the skin and strengthen the Guardian Qi shield covering your body.

In Nei Dan Qigong training, when you have filled up the Qi in these two vessels and can effectively circulate the Qi in them, you have achieved the "Small Circulation." In order to do this, you must know how to convert the essence stored in the kidneys into Qi, circulate this Qi in the Governing and Conception vessels, and finally lead this Qi to the head to nourish the brain and Shen (spirit).

2.   The Conception Vessel (Ren Mai)(Figure 2-26)
A.   Course:
Course #1:

(1). Lower abdomen below Qugu (Co-2) - (2). Ascends along the Midline of the abdomen and chest - (3). Crosses the throat and jaw - (4). winds around the mouth - (5). Terminates in the region of the eye.

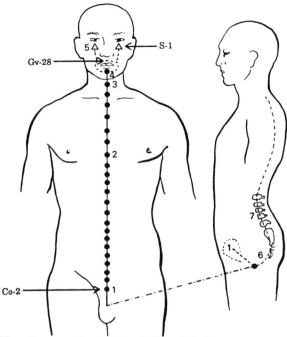

Figure 2-26. The Conception Vessel (Ren Mai).

Course #2:

(6). Pelvic cavity - (7). Enters the spine and ascends along the back.

***This vessel intersects Chengqi (S-1) and Yinjiao (Gv-28).

B. Cavities:

Huiyin (Co-1), Qugu (Co-2), Zhongli (Co-3), Guanyuan (Co-4), Shimen (Co-5), Qihai (Co-6), Abdomen-Yinjiao (Co-7), Shenjue (Co-8), Shuifen (Co-9), Xiawan (Co-10), Jianli (Co-11), Zhongwan (Co-12), Shangwan (Co-13), Juque (Co-14), Jiuwei (Co-15), Zhongting (Co-16), Shanzhong (Co-17), Yutang (Co-18), Chest-Zigong (Co-19), Huagai (Co-20), Xuanji (Co-21), Tiantu (Co-22), Lianquan (Co-23), and Chengjiang (Co-24).

C. Discussion:

Ren in Chinese means "direction, responsibility." Ren Mai, the "Conception Vessel," has a major role in Qi circulation, monitoring and directing all of the Yin channels (plus the stomach channel). The Conception Vessel is connected to the Thrusting and Yin Linking vessels, and is able to increase the Yin energy of the body.

This vessel nourishes the uterus (one of the five ancestral organs) and the whole genital system. It is said in the Nei Jing that the Conception and Thrusting vessels contain both blood and essence (Jing), and both flow up to the face and around the mouth. They contain more blood than essence in men, and thus promote the growth of the beard and body hair. Because women lose blood with their menstruation, they contain proportionately less blood and hence, no beard or body hair.

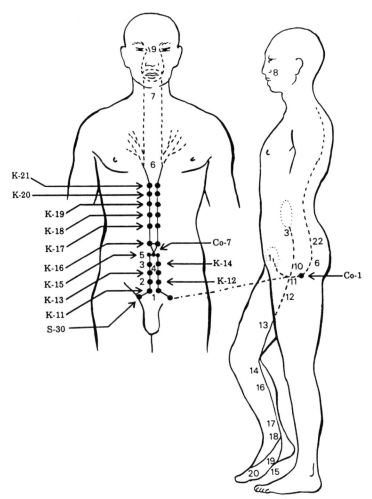

Figure 2-27. The Thrusting Vessel (Chong Mai).

It was described in the Su Wen that both the Conception and Thrusting vessels control the life cycles every 7 years for women and every 8 years for men. It is the changes taking place in these vessels at those intervals that promote the major alterations in our lives.

In addition, the Conception vessel also controls the distribution and "dispersion" of Guardian Qi all over the abdomen and thorax via numerous small Qi branches (Luo). This vessel also plays an important role in the distribution of body fluids in the abdomen.

In Qigong society, this vessel and the Governing vessel are considered the most important among the Qi channels and vessels, and must be trained first. It is believed that there is usually no significant Qi stagnation in the Conception vessel. However, it is important to increase the amount of Qi you are able to store, which also increases your ability to regulate the Yin channels.

3.   The Thrusting Vessel (Chong Mai)(Figure 2-27)
A.   Course:
Course #1:
(1). Lower abdomen - (2). Emerges along the Path of Qi - (3).

Tracks the course of the kidney channel - (4). Ascends through the abdomen - (5). Skirts the navel - (6). Disperses in the chest.

Course #2:

(6). Chest - (7). Ascends across the throat - (8). Face - (9). Nasal cavity.

Course #3:

(1). Lower abdomen - (10). Below the kidney - (11). Emerges along the Path of Qi - (12). Descends along the medial aspect of the thigh - (13). Popliteal fossa - (14). Medial margin of the tibia and the posterior aspect of the medial malleolus - (15). Bottom of the foot.

Course #4:

(16). Tibia - (17). Toward the lateral margin of the bone - (18). enters the heel - (19). Crosses the tarsal bones of the foot - (20). Big toe.

Course #5:

(21). Pelvic cavity - (22). Enter the spine and circulates through the back.

***This vessel intersects Huiyin (Co-1), Yinjiao (Co-7), Qichong (S-30), Henggu (K-11), Dahe (K-12), Qixue (K-13), Siman (K-14), Zhongzhu (K-15), Huangshu (K-16), Shangqu (K-17), Shiguan (K-18), Yindu (K-19), Tonggu (K-20), and Youmen (K-21).

B. Discussion:

One of the major purposes of the Thrusting vessel is to connect, to communicate, and to mutually support the Conception vessel. Because of this mutual Qi support, both can effectively regulate the Qi in the kidney channel. The kidneys are the residence of Original Qi and are considered one of the most vital Yin organs.

The Thrusting vessel is considered one of the most important and decisive vessels in successful Qigong training, especially in Marrow Washing. There are many reason for this. The first reason is that this vessel intersects two cavities on the Conception vessel: Huiyin (Co-1) and Yinjiao (Co-7). Huiyin means "meeting with Yin" and is the cavity where the Yang and Yin Qi are transferred. Yinjiao means "Yin Junction" and is the cavity where the Original Qi (Water Qi, or Yin Qi) interfaces with the Fire Qi created from food and air. The Thrusting Vessel also connects with eleven cavities on the kidney channel. The kidney is considered the residence of Original Essence (Yuan Jing), which is converted into Original Qi (Yuan Qi).

The second reason for the importance of the Thrusting Vessel in Qigong training is that this vessel is connected directly to the spinal cord and reaches up to the brain. The major goal of Marrow Washing Qigong is to lead the Qi into the marrow and then further on to the head, nourishing the brain and spirit (Shen).

And finally, the third reason is found in actual Qigong practice. There are three common training paths: Fire, Wind, and Water. In Fire path Qigong, the emphasis is on the Fire or Yang Qi circulating in the Governing vessel and therefore strengthening the muscles and

Figure 2-28. The Girdle Vessel (Dai Mai).

organs. The Fire path is the main Qi training in Muscle/Tendon Changing (Yi Jin Jing) Qigong. However, the Fire path can also cause the body to become too Yang, and therefore speed up the process of degeneration. In order to adjust the Fire to a proper level, Marrow Washing Qigong is also trained. This uses the Water path, in which Qi separates from the route of the Fire path at the Huiyin cavity (Co-1), enters the spinal cord, and finally reaches up to the head. The Water path teaches how to use Original Qi to cool down the body, and then to use this Qi to nourish the brain and train the spirit. Learning to adjust the Fire and Water Qi circulation in the body is called Kan-Li, which means Water-Fire. You can see from this that the Thrusting vessel plays a very important role in Qigong training.

4.   The Girdle Vessel (Dai Mai)(Figure 2-28)
A.   Course:

(1). Below the hypochondrium at the level of the 2nd lumbar vertebra - (2). Turns downward and encircles the body at the waist like a girdle.

***This vessel intersects Daimai (GB-26), Wushu (GB-27), and Weidao (GB-28).

B. Discussion:

The major purpose of the Girdle vessel is to regulate the Qi of the gall bladder. It is also responsible for the Qi's horizontal balance. If you have lost this balance, you will have lost your center and balance both mentally and physically.

From the point of view of Qigong, the Girdle vessel is also responsible for the strength of the waist area. When Qi is full and circulating smoothly, back pain will be avoided. In addition, because the kidneys are located nearby, this vessel is also responsible for Qi circulation around the kidneys, maintaining the kidneys' health. Most important of all for the Girdle vessel is the fact that the Lower Dan Tian is located in its area. In order to lead Original Qi from the kidneys to the Lower Dan Tian, the waist area must be healthy and relaxed. This means that the Qi flow in the waist area must be smooth. The training of the Girdle vessel has been highly developed, and will be discussed in a later YMAA Book.

5. The Yang Heel Vessel (Yangqiao Mai)(Figure 2-29)
A. Course:

(1). Below the lateral malleolus at Shenmai (B-62) - (2). Ascends along the lateral aspect of the leg - (3). Posterior aspect of the hypochondrium - (3). Lateral side of the shoulder - (4). Traverses the neck - (5). Passes beside the mouth - (6). Inner canthus (joins the Yin Heel vessel and the urinary bladder channel) - (7). Ascends across the forehead - (8). Winds behind the ear to Fengchi (GB-20) - (9). Enters the brain at Fengfu (Gv-16).

***This vessel intersects Shenmai (B-62), Pushen (B-61), Fuyang (B-59), Jingming (B-1), Juliao (GB-29), Fengchi (GB-20), Naoshu (SI-10), Jugu (LI-16), Jianyu (LI-15), Dicang (S-4), Juliao (S-3), Chengqi (S-1), and Fengfu (Gv-16).

B. Discussion:

While the preceding four vessels (Governing, Conception, Thrusting, and Girdle) are located in the trunk, the Yang Heel Vessel and the next three are located in the trunk and legs. (In addition, each of these four vessels is paired.) For millions of years, man has been walking on his legs, which preform much more strenuous work than the arms. I believe that it was because of this that, as evolution proceeded, the legs gradually developed these vessels to supply Qi support and regulate the channels. If this is true, it may be that, as time goes on and man uses his legs less and less, in a few million years these vessels will gradually disappear.

You can see from the way that the Yang Heel vessel intersects with other Qi channels that it regulates the Yang channels, such as the urinary bladder, the gall bladder, the small intestine, and the

Figure 2-29. The Yang Heel Vessel (Yangchiao Mai) and the Yin Heel Vessel (Yinchiao Mai).

large intestine. The Yang Heel vessel is also connected with the Governing vessel. The Qi filling this vessel is supplied mainly through exercising the legs, which converts the food essence or fat stored in the legs. This Qi is then led upward to nourish the Yang channels. It is believed in Qigong that, since this vessel is also connected with your brain, certain leg exercises can be used to cure headaches. Since a headache is caused by excess Qi in the head, exercising the legs will draw this Qi downward to the leg muscles and relieve the pressure in the head.

Most of the training that relates to this vessel is Wai Dan. Wai Dan Qigong is considered Yang, and specializes in training the Yang channels, while Nei Dan Qigong is considered relatively Yin and emphasizes the Yin channels more.

6. The Yin Heel Vessel (Yinqiao Mai)(Figure 2-29)
A. Course:

(1). Zhaohai (K-6) below the medial malleolus - (2). Extends upward along the medial aspect of the leg - (3). Crossing the perineum and chest entering the supraclavicular fossa - (4). Ascends through the throat and emerges in front of Renying (S-9) - (5). Traverses the medial aspect of the cheek - (6). Inner canthus (joins the urinary bladder channel and Yang Heel vessels) - (7). Ascends over the head and into the brain.

***This vessel intersects Zhaohai (K-6), Jiaoxin (K-8), and Jingming (B-1).

B. Discussion:
The Yin Heel vessel is connected with two cavities of the kidney channel. Therefore, one of the major sources of Qi for this vessel is the conversion of the kidney essence into Qi. It is believed in Qigong society that the other major Qi source is the essence of the external kidneys (testicles). In Marrow Washing Qigong, one of the training processes is to stimulate the testicles in order to increase the hormone production and increase the conversion of the essence into Qi. At the same time, you would learn how to lead the Qi in this vessel up to the head to nourish the brain and spirit (Shen). With this nourishment, you would be able to reach Buddhahood or enlightenment. From a health and longevity point of view, the raised spirit will be able to efficiently direct the Qi of the entire body and maintain your health.

7. The Yang Linking Vessel (Yangwei Mai)(Figure 2-30)
A. Course:
(1). Jinmen (B-63) on the heel - (2). Ascends along the lateral aspect of the leg - (3). Lower abdomen - (4). Slants upward across the posterior aspect of the hypochondrium - (5). Across the posterior axillary fold to the shoulder - (6). Ascends the neck and crosses behind the ear - (7). Proceeds to the forehead - (8). Doubles back over the head - (9). Fengfu (Gv-16).

***This vessel intersects Jinmen (B-63), Yangjiao (GB-35), Jianjing (GB-21), Fengchi (GB-20), Naokong (GB-19), Chengling (GB-18), Zhengying (GB-17), Muchuang (GB-16), Head-Linqi (GB-15), Yangbai (GB-14), Benshen (GB-13), Tianliao (TB-15), Naoshu (SI-10), Yamen (Gv-15), Fengfu (Gv-16), and Touwei (S-8).

B. Discussion:
The Yang Linking vessel regulates the Qi mainly in the Yang channels: the urinary bladder, gall bladder, triple burner, small intestine, and stomach channels. It is also connected with the Governing vessel at Yamen (Gv-15) and Fengfu (Gv-16). This vessel and the Yang Heel vessel have not been emphasized much in Qigong, except in Iron Shirt training where these two and the Governing vessel are trained.

8. The Yin Linking Vessel (Yinwei Mai)(Figure 2-30)
A. Course:
(1). Lower leg at Zhubin (K-9) - (2). Ascending along the medial aspect of the leg - (3). Enters the lower abdomen - (4). Upward across

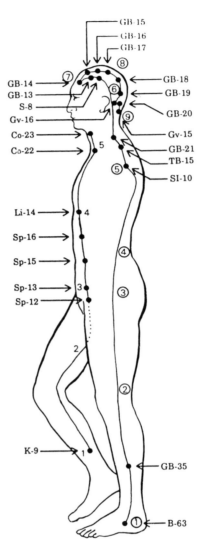

Figure 2-30. The Yang Linking Vessel (Yangwei Mai) and the Yin Linking Vessel (Yinwei Mai).

the chest - (5). Throat (meets Tiantu (Co-22) and Lianquan (Co-23)).

***This vessel intersects Zhubin (K-9), Chongmen (Sp-12), Fushe (Sp-13), Daheng (Sp-15), Fuai (Sp-16), Qimen (Li-14), Tiantu (Co-22), and Lianquan (Co-23).

B. Discussion:
The Yin Linking vessel has connections with the kidney, spleen, and liver Yin channels. The Yin Linking vessel also communicates with the Conception vessel at two cavities. This vessel is not trained much in Qigong.

2-4. Understanding the Mental Body
Let us now discuss the third part of the human body, the mental or spiritual body. First, let us consider the difference between the

mental and the spiritual. Even with today's science, it is very difficult to define these two aspects of our nature, so we must look to the experiences gained in the past. According to Chinese understanding, the mental part of us includes both the physical and the Qi aspects of our being which are related to thinking. The physical parts are the nervous system and the brain, which need Qi to exist and function. If the physical brain and nervous system receive the right amount of Qi and stay healthy, the mind will be able to think clearly and judge wisely. However, if the Qi supply is not normal, the brain and nervous system will not function properly, and mental problems may occur. Naturally, if the Qi supply stops, these physical systems will die. Therefore, in order to keep the mental system functioning properly, Chinese Qigong places heavy emphasis on learning how to lead Qi to the brain to nourish it, and also how to maintain the entire nervous system.

Only when the mental aspect of your being is healthy are you able to build up the spiritual part of your body. It is very difficult to understand and define this spiritual part. The various religions were created to search for the truth of this matter. Asian religions believe that when the human spirit has been cultivated to a very high level, we will be able to leave the cycle of reincarnation and gain eternal life. Religions in the West have similar beliefs.

The mental part of our being can be considered a lower level of our spirit which has not yet been well cultivated. The Chinese religions believe that when this lower level of spirit is cultivated, the Qi in the body will be able to combine and communicate with the Qi of nature. This enables us to better understand the patterns of natural Qi, and ultimately learn how to avoid reincarnation and gain spiritual independence. This level of growth is called "enlightenment" in Daoism and "Buddhahood" in Buddhism.

The mental part of our being is actually our thinking, which can be manifested externally. When manifestation occurs, the process is completed through the Qi circulatory and nervous systems. This means that the mind, Qi, and physical body cannot be separated. In order to calm down the physical body, we must first calm down the Qi body through the nervous system. In order to calm down the Qi body, we must first regulate the mind.

Because of the closeness of the mind, Qi, and physical body, regulating the mind is an important part of Qigong training. Chinese medicine and Qigong teach that there are two minds, one is called "Xin" and the other is called "Yi." The mind which is generated by emotional disturbances is called "Xin." Xin means "heart" in Chinese. Any occurrence which is able to touch your heart and disturb your neutral mind is called "Xin." For example, if you are upset because someone has said something bad about you, the thoughts or intentions that you have are considered to be Xin. Or when your regular Qigong practice time comes by, but you are lazy and decide not to practice, the thinking which led to this decision is called Xin. "Xin" can therefore be translated "emotional mind."

However, when the thoughts come from wise thinking and clear judgement, then this kind of mind is called "Yi," which can be translated as "intention" or "wisdom mind." What the wisdom mind has conceived, you can usually accomplish.

Unfortunately, the emotional mind usually dominates the wisdom mind. When people react to events, it is usually according to their emotional feelings rather than their calm judgement. One of the main goals of Chinese Qigong is developing the wisdom mind so that it can "govern" the emotional mind. When this happens, emotional disturbances will not occur, and the mind can be peaceful and calm. The emotional mind is considered to be Yang while the wisdom mind is Yin. The training works to balance Yin and Yang.

You can see that the mental body actually is constructed of two "minds." When either mind is too strong and causes your actions to deviate from the neutral, balanced state, you then lose your mental balance. This will also affect how your physical body functions. According to Chinese religious Qigong, when the Yin and Yang minds are in mutual balance, the human spirit can be raised to a supernatural state and reach the stage of enlightenment or Buddhahood.

In general massage, to relax the physical body you must first remove emotional disturbances from the mind. This means that the first thing you should do is to massage the mental body so that the mind can be calm and relaxed. Only when the patient's mind is relaxed can their physical body be relaxed. Only when the physical body is relaxed can the Qi move easily and smoothly in the body. This is the key to successful massage.

2-5. Gates and Junctions in the Human Body

In this section, we would like to explain two terms which are used frequently in Qigong. The first term is "Men," which can be translated "gate" or "door;" the second term is "Jie," which can be translated "knot" or "junction."

A "gate" usually means a door through which the Qi can enter or exit a place. They are therefore commonly called "Qi gates." Actually, in Chinese medicine, these gates are called "Qi Xue" (Qi cavities) or simply "Xue" (cavities). According to Chinese medicine and Qigong, many of these Qi gates are crucial in maintaining health, curing sicknesses, and even practicing Qigong. These gates are usually called "Qiao Men" (tricky gates) in order to distinguish them from the other gates. Most of these gates are used in Qigong massage. Since obstructions in these gates can affect the smooth circulation of Qi, treating them properly can improve the Qi circulation.

Many of these tricky gates have several different names which are used by the various groups that utilize them. Names may vary between the physicians, martial artists, Qigong practitioners, and the religious communities. For example, the cavity between the thumb and the second finger is called "Hegu" in medicine, while it is

Figure 2-31. The Laogong cavity (P-8).

called "Hukou" in martial arts society. The cavity on the top of the head is called "Baihui" in medicine, "Tianlingai" in the martial arts, and "Niwangong" in Daoist Qigong. Therefore, do not be confused if you hear someone call a cavity by a different name.

There are two types of gates. One is the "external Qi gate," through which Qi can enter or leave the body. You can use these gates to adjust the body's energy level. For example, when you are excited or nervous, your heart has an excess of "fire," which may damage it. The excess heat in the heart can be moved to the pericardium, and then brought through the Qi channels to the center of the palms, where it can be released into the air through the Laogong cavities (Figure 2-31). When this happens, your palms feel warm and perspire.

The communication of Qi between your body and the air does not happen only through the acupuncture cavities. There are many non-cavity gates, such as the nose and anus, which handle a great deal of the work.

The second type of Qi gate is the "internal Qi gate," which enables the Qi to communicate between the different parts of the body. Many of these gates are cavities, while many others are not. For example, the neck is the Qi gate through which the head and the body communicate. The joints in the arms and legs are also considered gates.

The second term you need to understand is "Jie," which means "knot" or "junction." Usually the term refers to physical knots or junctions, such as where a large nerve or blood vessel branches out into many smaller nerves or vessels. When these areas are tense, they can interfere with smooth Qi and blood circulation. Most of these places are also Qi gates, which is not surprising, since it is the Qi which controls the nervous system.

In this section, we will first discuss the gates on the surface of the body, and then we will identify others which are inside the body. We will only mention the more important gates here. Others will be discussed in the appropriate sections when we discuss general massage in Part Two.

Gates on the Surface of the Body:

1.   Eyes, Mouth, Ears, and Nose:

These four organs are the most important gates which allow you to communicate with the outside world. Whenever you look at something, your eyes receive energy (Qi) from it, and this energy is passed to your brain for recognition. The eyes are usually considered to only receive Qi, although many Qigong masters believe that the eyes can also emit it.

The mouth takes in food, which Chinese medicine and Qigong consider to be "Post-birth essence." It is this essence, when it is converted into Qi, which nourishes the body. Therefore, the main purpose of the mouth is to receive this essence. However, when you are sick, the mouth is also used to release extra heat or waste from the body. For example, when you have a cold, coughing releases heat. The sounds which come out of the mouth can also release Qi from the body, and different sounds can release the excess Qi from different organs. For example, when you are happy your heart has an excess of "fire" or heat. When you laugh you make the sound "Ha," which releases the heat. The mouth plays an important part in Qigong, and a great deal of study has been devoted to how different sounds can be used to balance the Qi in the internal organs.

The ears receive sound energy, and the brain responds to the different wavelengths of the energy. Like the eyes, the ears are not normally used to release or emit energy.

Finally, the nose brings air into and out of the body. When you inhale, you take in oxygen, another form of "Post-birth essence, which is converted into Qi. The nose also releases carbon-dioxide which we do not need in the body. Chemically, when the oxygen is taken into the body, a chemical reaction begins. The final product of this reaction is carbon-dioxide, which contains the body's waste carbon (from the biochemical reaction). This is eliminated from your body when you exhale.

2.   Anus and Urethra:

The anus and urethra are also gates which release waste from the body, and, at the same time, release excess Qi. When waste elimination is irregular, your body can be in a state of either excess or deficiency. For instance, when you have diarrhea your body becomes deficient because of the too frequent elimination, but when you are constipated, there will be an excess of Qi in your body, and you will feel heat accumulating internally. Because of this, both Western and oriental physicians will check their patient's regularity as a part of their diagnosis. The same theory also applies to the urethra.

3.   Pores:

The millions of pores in your skin are probably responsible for releasing the greatest amount of Qi from your body. When you are too hot, the heat is released through the pores. In the summertime, when the Qi in your internal organs is normally sufficient, and the Qi in the surrounding air is also sufficient, your pores will be wide open to release any excess heat from your body. However, in the wintertime, the Qi in the surrounding air is deficient. In order to protect your internal Qi, most of your pores will stay closed to seal the Qi inside. You can see that your pores are designed to adjust the Qi in the body.

An important part of Chinese Qigong is the practice of skin breathing. This makes it possible for the Qi to reach all the pores smoothly so that they can keep functioning properly. Naturally, the activity of the pores is controlled by the sensations you receive from the nerves in your skin. You can keep the nervous system functioning properly if you keep it supplied with a steady amount of Qi. It is believed that the most effective way of preventing colds is to practice "skin breathing" Qigong. This technique is discussed in the YMAA book "The Root of Chinese Chi Kung."

There is another Qigong practice in which Qi can be stored in the bone marrow instead of being released into the air and wasted. This practice is called "Brain/Marrow Washing Qigong." Normally, aging is caused by deficient Qi nourishment of the brain and of the bone marrow, which manufactures blood cells. If Qi can be led inward to the brain and bone marrow, they can keep functioning significantly longer than usual. In addition, the excess Qi produced in the body can be efficiently used, instead of released into the air. Conserving Qi is especially important as you get older; in fact, it is the key to longevity. If you would like to know more about brain/marrow washing Qigong, please refer to the YMAA book "Muscle/Tendon Changing and Marrow/Brain Washing Chi Kung."

4. Tips of Fingers and Toes:

According to Chinese medicine, there are six primary Qi channels connected to the tips of the fingers, and another six connected to the tips of the toes. It is believed that because we are continually using the fingers for working and the toes for walking, the Qi has to reach smoothly to the tips of the fingers and toes to maintain their sensitivity. This is the reason for the gates in the ends of the toes and fingers. These gates are the reason that, when you massage someone with your fingers, you can exchange Qi effectively with them.

5. Cavities:

It has recently been discovered that what Chinese acupuncture calls cavities are actually tiny spots of higher electrical conductivity than the surrounding skin.(*1) This higher conductivity creates a tunnel or path from the surface to the primary Qi channels under the skin and muscles (Figure 2-32). The cavities bring the excess Qi circulating in the primary Qi channels out to the surface of the skin and release it to the air. All of these cavities can be used in Qigong massage to release excess Qi.

Of the more than 700 acupuncture cavities, about 108 can be reached by the fingers. Acupressure and Dian Xue are systems of

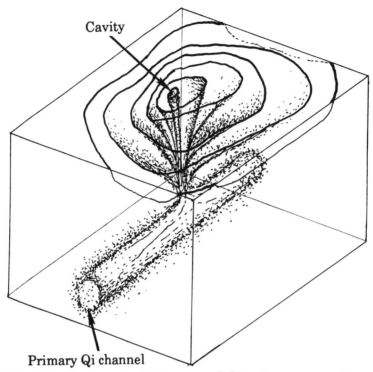

Cavity

Primary Qi channel

Figure 2-32. Electrical conductivity map of skin at an acupuncture point.

treatment which use the hands or fingers to press and rub the cavities in order to regulate the Qi circulation in the channels. Some of the Dian Xue techniques are well known and used frequently by practitioners of general massage.

A number of the cavities are larger than the others, and it is easier to establish communication with the Qi through them. These cavities play an important role in Qigong massage. These gates are the Baihui, Naohu, Yintang, Mingmen, Laogong, and Yongquan cavities. The most important of these are the two Laogong cavities located in the centers of the palms (Figure 2-33), and the two Yongquan cavities located on the bottom of the feet (Figure 2-34). These four gates are used to regulate the condition of the Qi in the heart and the kidneys. Massaging these four gates keeps them open and exchanging Qi with the environment.

There are a few other gates or areas through which the Qi can communicate easily inside and outside of the body. For example, the nipples are considered Qi gates, although they have not been studied very extensively. Also, the pores around the joints are more open than elsewhere, and so the Qi exchange occurs there more easily.

Gates or Junctions Inside the Body:
1. Joint Junctions:

Joints are the junctions or passages where the Qi and blood communicate between one section of the body and another. If the Qi and blood circulation is blocked at a joint, a part of the body will not

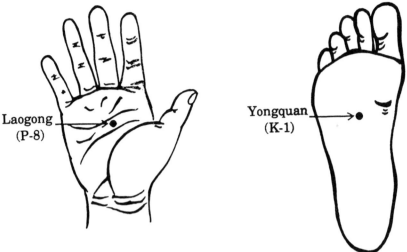

Figure 2-33. The Laogong cavity.

Figure 2-34. The Yongquan cavity.

obtain the proper nourishment, and will malfunction or suffer some damage as a consequence.

In Qigong massage, the joints are separated into three categories. The first category consists of the central joints (i.e., spinal joints) which are the passageway for Qi and neural messages between the brain and every part of the body. Since these joints are related to our thinking and feeling, they are considered to be the most important in Qigong massage. The second most important set of joints are those which connect the six major parts of the body. These six parts are the head, the two arms, the two legs, and the torso. These six main parts are connected by the neck, the shoulder joints, and the hip joints. The third kind of junction includes all the other joints of the body. Although some are more important than others, they are all junctions of Qi and blood. These joints include the jaw, elbows, wrists, finger joints, knees, ankles, toe joints, and a number of other, minor ones.

Whenever you are tense, the Qi and the blood circulation in the joints can be affected. Blockages of the joint junctions can also have many other causes, such as injuries, joint diseases such as arthritis, degeneration due to aging, etc. In massage, when you have loosened the joints, you are already one third of the way to your goal.

2. Junctions of the Arteries and Nerves:

The body contains many nerve and artery junctions, usually where a main artery or nerve branches out into many smaller arteries or nerves. An example is the place under the ear where the main artery and nerves branch upward from the neck (Figure 2-35). Whenever this place is blocked, the brain will not obtain enough oxygen, and brain cells will wither or even die. You therefore need to learn how to massage this area to keep the junction open. Although many junctions are located around the joints, many other are not related to the joints (e.g., the temple).

Figure 2-35. Anatomical structure of the head.

3. Gates to the Main Nerves:

We have already explained how, in Qigong, the nervous system, mind, and Qi cannot be separated. Since the nerves are the bridge between the mind and the Qi, Qigong massage devotes a great deal of attention to massaging the nerves.

In addition to massaging the nerve endings such as are found in the skin, general massage also has ways to massage the major nerves. There are many places in the body where you can reach them. These gates are usually found on the Yin sides of the joints, such as on the inside of the elbows (Figure 2-36), the back of the knees, and in the armpits. Since these gates access the central nervous system, it is important to use the correct techniques and the proper amount of power. Too much stimulation will only cause more tension, and increase Qi and blood stagnation.

4. Qi Junctions:

There are twelve primary Qi channels in the body. The Qi circulating in them can be affected by our thinking, tension, sickness, or by the food and air we take in. There are a number of places where the Qi is most likely to become stagnant. Most of these places are also where the acupuncture cavities are located. Physicians can insert a needle through the cavity to reach the stagnation and

Figure 2-36. Anatomical structure of the arm.

release it, or else they can massage the area and release the stagnation. In fact, this is how Dian Xue massage treats illness.

When you study Qigong massage, you must learn the paths of the twelve channels, as well as which places are likely to become stagnant, and how to remove the stagnation by stimulating the cavities.

Chinese medicine and Qigong consider the junctions where a channel or vessel with Yin Qi joins a channel or vessel with Yang Qi (or vice versa) to be extremely important for your health. It is believed that when the Qi cannot transmit smoothly from one phase to another, you may become sick. Usually, these transmissions or changes happen according to natural timing, such as the transition between day and night, the lunar month, the seasons, or the year. For example, the Qi is circulating more strongly in the front (Yin) side of your body during the daytime, and in the back (Yang) side of your body during the night.

In general Qigong massage, there are two cavities which are considered the most important for the exchange of Yin and Yang. The first one is the Huiyin cavity, located in the perineum between

Huiyin (Co-1)

Figure 2-37. The Huiyin cavity (Co-1).

Renzhong (Gv-26)

Figure 2-38. The Renzhong cavity (Gv-26).

the genitals and anus (Figure 2-37). The Huiyin cavity is the place where the Yin Conception Vessel joins the Yang Governing Vessel.

The second cavity is called Renzhong, and is located under the nose (Figure 2-38). Although this cavity is not the exact location where the Yin-Yang exchange takes place (which is actually in the roof of the mouth), stimulating this cavity will improve the exchange.

In addition to regulating the transmission of Qi, these two cavities can also be used to raise up the spirit of vitality, for example, in reviving someone who has fainted.

2-6. Important Points in Qigong Massage

Whichever type of Qigong massage you are practicing, there are a number of important points which you should keep in mind:

1. The temperature in the room should be warm enough so that the patient is comfortable. During the massage, their body will be wholly or partially exposed to the air. If it is too cold, they may be tense, and they may even catch a cold. Needless to say, this would prevent you from gaining their whole-hearted cooperation.

2. You should use a massage table which is comfortable for the patient, and of a height which is comfortable for you. If the table is too high or too low, it will feel awkward to you, and your concentration will be disturbed.

3. The patient should dress comfortably, with loose clothing. Also, whatever they are lying on should be made of natural material. For example, if they are lying on polyester sheet, a great mass of Qi (static charges) can accumulate in the material and affect the treatment.

4. The air should be circulating gently. If the air is stagnant, both you and the patient will feel uncomfortable.

5. Do not massage a person who has just eaten, or who is hungry, since the massage might be uncomfortable, especially when you work on their stomach.

6. Don't have a light directly over the patient, since this would make them uncomfortable.

7. The room should be as quiet as possible. Noise is always disturbing during massage, though sometimes soft music might help them to relax.

8. The patient's body should be clean, and your hands should also be clean and warm. Many masseurs will place a silk handkerchief on the area they are massaging to avoid directly touching the skin. However, this reduces the sensitivity of their touch, and limits the Qi communication between them and the patient.

9. Before starting, always ask yourself the following questions. What is the purpose of the massage? What does the patient expect? Is the massage for relaxation and enjoyment, or is it to treat an illness? Am I confident that I have enough experience to give this massage? Remember, understanding yourself and the patient is the key to a successful treatment.

10. Always understand the patient's body. Different levels of power should be used for different patients, and for different purposes. You will also vary the techniques you use, depending upon the

patient. The better you understand the patient's body, the more you will know about the battlefield upon which you are fighting sickness.

11. Always diagnose the case carefully, and determine how serious the problem is. For example, if the injury involves a cracked bone, then you should not massage the area with power, since that would hinder the healing of the bone. Wrong treatments only make matters worse.

12. When you massage a patient, do not cause pain or tickle them, since this will cause them to tense.

13. If you are treating the patient externally with herbs, do not apply them anywhere where there are cuts or breaks in the skin, since this may cause an infection.

14. Keep your fingernails short! Long nails will limit how you can use your hands, and they will make your patient nervous.

15. You must reach an understanding with your patient if you are to massage any area about which they are shy.

16. Ask the patient for permission before using massage oil. Some people don't like it.

17. Always explain to the patient or massage partner what you are going to do. This will allow them to prepare themselves mentally, and will increase their confidence in you.

Reference

(*1). "The Body Electric" by Robert O. Becker, M.D. and Gary Selden, Quill, William Morrow, New York, 1985.

Chapter 3
Massage Techniques

3-1. Introduction

Before going into the specific practices of each category of massage, we would like to first introduce the most common techniques. Using the correct techniques will help you to treat problems effectively, while using the wrong techniques will often make matters worse. It is difficult to make general statements about what techniques you should use to treat particular problems, since what works well on one person may not work as well on another. Furthermore, even with the same technique, you may use a different amount of power with each person. One person may be extremely sensitive in a particular area, while another person may not feel any but your strongest power. Experience is your greatest teacher. The more people you massage, the easier it will be for you to determine what needs to be done.

In this chapter, we will introduce many techniques. Over the years, many other techniques have been developed. However, because space is limited, and because some of the techniques have very specific uses, we will not be able to list them all. This chapter is meant to serve as a reference, and to give you guidelines for how to approach massage.

In the next section we will introduce the parts of the body that you will use in giving a massage, and in section 3-3 we will discuss the techniques.

3-2. The Tools of Massage

Everyone knows that various areas of the hands are used in massage. However, many other parts of the body can also be used, such as the elbows, the forearms, and the heels.

1.   Finger Tips:

A fingertip covers a very small area, so its power can usually penetrate deep. Because of this, the fingertips are usually used to

Figure 3-1.

Figure 3-2.

Figure 3-3.

Figure 3-4.

treat injuries deep inside the body, or to stimulate circulation in the primary Qi channels.

In Tui Na massage, you usually rub with one or more fingertips when the injured area is small or deep, such as at particular points in the wrist, back of hand, or in the palm between the bases of the fingers (Figure 3-1). You would also use one or more fingertips to press inward on the skin and push along the Qi channels (Figure 3-2). The tips of the thumb, index finger, and sometimes the middle finger are used.

In Dian Xue massage, the fingertip is also commonly used for pressing, usually together with vibrating or shaking. To do this, you place your fingertip on the appropriate cavity, and then concentrate your mind so that your power reaches the Qi primary channel to either stimulate or soothe the Qi. Dian Xue usually uses the tip of the thumb (Figure 3-3) or the second finger (Figure 3-4). Sometimes

Figure 3-5.

Figure 3-6.

Figure 3-7.

Figure 3-8.

the tip of the middle finger is also used (Figure 3-5). Since the Qi primary channel in the middle finger is connected to the pericardium, which is related to the heart, the Qi is usually strongest there.

In addition, since the fingertips are also Qi gates, they are often used in Qi massage to trace the Qi channels to adjust the circulation. This is usually done with the "sword secret" hand form (Figure 3-6). Sometimes only the middle finger is used (Figure 3-7). When fingertips are used for Qi massage, they either touch the skin very lightly, or not at all.

In relaxation or general massage, the fingertips are commonly used to tap and stimulate the skin (Figure 3-8), which relaxes the patient and brings stagnant Qi to the surface.

2. The Last Section of the Fingers:

The last section of the fingers is the part most commonly used for rubbing and pressing. It covers a larger area than the fingertip does, and so a massage with it is gentler and softer than with the fingertip.

Figure 3-9.

Figure 3-10.

Figure 3-11.

Figure 3-12.

In Tui Na massage, it is the most effective way of spreading out bruises and Qi stagnation so that waste material and stagnant Qi and/or blood can be removed. This is done by rubbing with a circular or straight motion. Usually, the last section of the thumb is used (Figure 3-9). However, the last sections of the index and middle fingers are also commonly used together for this purpose (Figure 3-10). These areas are also used to press and push along the Qi channels to adjust the Qi.

In Dian Xue massage, the last section of the fingers, especially of the thumb (Figure 3-11) and index finger (Figure 3-12), are commonly used for pressing cavities. This stimulates a larger area than a fingertip would, but it is the preferred method because it is not as painful for the patient. Since the patient stays more relaxed, recovery is quicker.

Figure 3-13.

Figure 3-14.

Figure 3-15.

Figure 3-16.

For relaxation or general massage, the last sections of the five fingers are used to adhere to the skin while using circular movements to relax an area (Figure 3-13). Sometimes, the last section of the thumb (Figure 3-14), or index and middle fingers (Figure 3-15), is used to rub a smaller area to disperse acid which has accumulated in the muscles and tendons.

3.   The Last Two Sections of the Fingers:

The last two sections of the fingers are commonly used to grab muscles or tendons for Tui Na massage and relaxation massage. Usually, all five fingers are used at the same time. They are mainly used to massage the muscles on the limbs, such as on the arms (Figure 3-16), thighs (Figure 3-17), and calves (Figure 3-18). They are also often used to massage the big muscles, such as the muscles beside the armpit (Figure 3-19), and the muscles between the neck and shoulders (Figure 3-20).

Figure 3-17.

Figure 3-18.

Figure 3-19.

Figure 3-20.

This type of massage is usually used to spread out stagnant Qi and blood, as well as to stimulate areas to relax the patient.

4.   Knuckles:

The knuckles are commonly used in Tui Na and Dian Xue massage, but only occasionally used in relaxation massage.

In Tui Na massage, the knuckle of the thumb (Figure 3-21) or the index finger (Figure 3-22) are normally used to press down and then push along the Qi channels to stimulate the Qi. Often, all of the knuckles except the thumb are used in a circular motion to massage areas where Qi and blood have become stagnate (Figure 3-23).

In Dian Xue massage, normally the knuckles of the thumb (Figure 3-24) or the index finger (Figure 3-25) are used to press inward through the cavities to stimulate the Qi circulation in the primary Qi channels. Quite often a vibrating motion will be used along with the pressure.

Figure 3-21.

Figure 3-22.

Figure 3-23.

Figure 3-24.

5. Side of the Palm:

The side of the palm is commonly used for Tui Na and relaxation massage. In Tui Na, after deep stimulation with other techniques, such as fingertip massage, has brought stagnant Qi and blood to the surface, then the side of the palm can be used to spread out the Qi and blood even more. The side of the palm covers a large area, and so it is used on large muscles on the torso or on joints such as the hip, knee, shoulder, or neck. The same techniques are also used in relaxation massage to spread acid accumulated in the muscles. The side of the palms are usually used for circular rubbing (Figure 3-26) and straight line pushing massage (Figure 3-27).

6. Base of the Palm:

Like the side of the palm, the base of the palm is used to cover a larger area in Tui Na and relaxation massage. The base of the palm is stronger than the side because you can use your body as the root

Figure 3-25.

Figure 3-26.

Figure 3-27.

Figure 3-28.

of the technique (Figure 3-28), whereas with the side of the palm you usually use your shoulder as the root.

The techniques for the base of the palm are the same as those for the side of the palm. However, there is one extra application for the base of the palm which is widely used, which is pressing without rubbing. This application is especially useful in loosening up the spine. It is done by pressing down on the joints between the vertebrae, one by one (Figure 3-29). This cannot be done easily with the side of the palm.

7. Center of the Palm:

In the center of each palm is a cavity or Qi gate called Laogong (Figure 3-30) which is used for dissipating extra heat in the heart.

Figure 3-29.

Figure 3-30. The Laogong cavity (P-8).

Figure 3-31.

The Laogong cavity is on the Qi channel of the pericardium, which is the sack or membrane around the heart. Whenever there is too much "fire" in the heart (i.e., when it is too Yang), the excess heat is conducted through the pericardium channel to the center of your palms. As long as you are healthy, the Qi in your heart is more positive than necessary, and the excess Qi is constantly being released through the Laogong cavities. This means that the Qi is stronger at the Laogong than elsewhere, and so this is the best cavity to use when you wish to lead a patient's Qi.

The center of the palm is commonly used for relaxation or general massage, as well as for Qi massage. In relaxation massage, the patient's Qi can be led while only lightly touching the skin (Figure 3-31) because the Qi released from your Laogong cavity can easily correspond with it. You only need to rub gently, and to let your hands flow soothingly on their skin to relax them and open them up to your treatment. The hand is your main tool for regulat-

Figure 3-32.

Figure 3-33.

Figure 3-34.

ing your patient's emotions, and therefore their Yi and Qi. If you can skillfully use your hands to bring your patient into a relaxed state, you have already completed 50% of the treatment.

In Qi massage, you use the Qi released from your Laogong to correspond with the Qi in the patient's body (Figure 3-32). This allows you to restore smooth, healthy circulation, and to remove Qi stagnation from injuries or other causes.

8. Forearm and Elbow:

The forearm and elbow are not used very often in massage, however, there are times when they can be very useful. The forearm can be used in relaxation massage for large muscles when the hand is not strong enough; for example, the trunk muscles on the back (Figure 3-33), or the thigh muscles (Figure 3-34). The forearm is sometimes used in Tui Na to spread out accumulated Qi and blood.

Figure 3-35.

Figure 3-36.

Figure 3-37.

Figure 3-38.

The elbow is sometimes used in Tui Na or Dian Xue massage because its power is stronger and more penetrating. It is used especially for cavities located in areas with big muscles, such as the hips and thighs (Figure 3-35).

9.   Knee and Bottom of Foot:

The knee and the bottom of the feet are often used by women and by men with small builds in both Chinese and Japanese massage. They are used mainly for the back, hips, and thighs (Figures 3-36, 3-37, and 3-38) where the muscles are especially thick and strong, and the masseur therefore needs strong hands if the power is to penetrate.

Figure 3-39.   Figure 3-40.

3-3. Massage Techniques and Training

In this section, we will introduce fifty basic massage techniques used in Chinese Qigong massage. Naturally, some of them are more effective for one category of massage than another. Once you have studied these techniques, you may discover others that are useful in some cases.

1. Rubbing (Rou or Mo)(揉，摩):

The Chinese word "Rou" is made up of the two characters "hand" (才) and "soft"(柔). This implies that the Rubbing technique massages or rubs softly with the hand. It also implies that the hand doing the technique should be "soft" or relaxed, with pressure coming from the whole body, guided by the relaxed and concentrated mind. There is no exact English word for this concept. "Mo" means almost the same thing, but implies a little larger movement, and includes some friction. Rou is generally a circular motion, while Mo is a straight, back and forth motion. In actual practice, there is almost no difference between the two.

Rubbing is the most common technique, and it can be used in general massage, Tui Na massage, and also Dian Xue massage. Naturally, although the theory and the basic movement are the same, the applications may be different in each category. For example, when Rubbing is used for an injury, it is used over a larger area because you want to get rid of local bruises and stagnant Qi. However, when Rubbing is used for healing illness, its power is focused on the primary channels or cavities to balance the Qi circulation. Also, the part of your hand you use for Rubbing will vary according to the application.

Rubbing is usually done with a circular motion. You may use the last section of your thumb (Figure 3-39), or the last section of one or more fingers (Figure 3-40), the last joint of the fingers (Figure 3-41), the side of the palm (Figure 3-42), base of the palm (Figure 3-43), or forearm (Figure 3-44).

Figure 3-41.

Figure 3-42.

Figure 3-43.

Figure 3-44.

When you use Rubbing, you do not actually rub the patient's skin. Instead, your hand contacts their skin and moves with it, so that you are actually rubbing under their skin. This lets you remove stagnant Qi and blood in the fascia between the skin and the muscles. Since your power is going beneath the skin, you can direct it to the muscles, the fascia between the muscles, or even to the fascia between the muscles and the bones.

Generally speaking, if you rub with your right hand in a clockwise direction (from your perspective), then you are releasing Qi to the patient. From the patient's perspective, your hand is moving counterclockwise, and the patient is absorbing the Qi (Figure 3-45). If you rub in a counterclockwise direction with your right hand, then you are absorbing Qi from the patient.

Rubbing is used to first relax the muscles or the injured area, and then to improve the Qi and blood circulation. Rubbing helps to

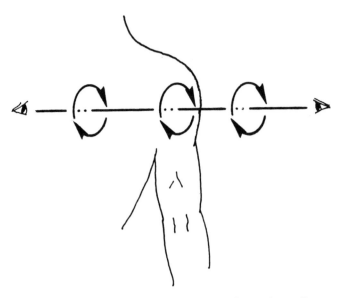

Figure 3-45. Different viewpoints for the direction of massage.

Figure 3-46.

Figure 3-47.

remove stagnant Qi and blood and bring them to the skin. Finally, Rubbing spreads the Qi and blood even farther so that the body can remove it. Rubbing is very effective in removing the acid which accumulates in the muscles when you exercise.

Tui Na massage is frequently used for joint injuries. Rubbing is used first to bring the Qi and bruise to the surface, and then circular and straight Rubbing (Figure 3-46) are used to push the stagnant Qi and blood away from the joint so that the body can take care of the residue.

In Dian Xue massage, the circular motion is very small. Normally, the first section of the finger is used to press down heavily on a cavity, then a small, circular rubbing motion is used to lead power into the cavity (Figure 3-47).

Figure 3-48.

Figure 3-49.

Figure 3-50.

Figure 3-51.

2. Pressing (An)(按):

Pressing straight inward is called "An." Pressing is often used together with other techniques. For example, in the Rubbing technique, Pressing is required to adjust the depth of the massage. Pressing can be applied through the fingertips (Figure 3-48), the last section of the fingers (Figure 3-49), the base of the palm (Figure 3-50), the forearm (Figure 3-51), or the elbow (Figure 3-52). Dian Xue massage normally uses Pressing with the fingertips and the last section of the fingers (especially the thumb and/or the index fingers)(Figure 3-53). In Tui Na or general massage, the base of the palm or the forearm are commonly used to press the spine, the trunk muscles, or even the kidneys.

In Dian Xue massage, you apply pressure with this technique and then release it. Doing this repeatedly stimulates the area or cavity and affects the Qi circulation there.

Figure 3-52.

Figure 3-53.

Figure 3-54.

Figure 3-55.

3. Pushing (Tui)(推):

Pushing combines Pressing with straight movements. It is normally used right after circular Rubbing. Pushing can be done with the last section of the fingers (especially the thumb)(Figure 3-54), the side of the palm (Figure 3-55), the base of the palm (Figure 3-56), or the forearm. Pushing can also be combined with other techniques such as Rubbing (Figure 3-57) or Vibrating.

Pushing is commonly used in both general and Tui Na massage. In general massage, Pushing is used to push and spread the acid accumulated in the muscles. In Tui Na massage, a straight pushing motion is used to spread bruises and Qi out away from the area of stagnation. The more the bruises and stagnant Qi are spread out, the easier it will be for the body's natural blood and Qi circulation to assist the healing. In general, you do not want the stagnation to be focused in a tiny area, because this is more difficult for the body's healing processes to handle.

Figure 3-56.   Figure 3-57.

Figure 3-58.   Figure 3-59.

4.   Grabbing (Na)(拿):

You can use Grabbing with one or both hands. Grabbing is used to stabilize a limb for pushing, to correct dislocated joints, or to connect broken bones (Figure 3-58). Grabbing is also used on the limbs for cavity press. The thumb presses on the cavity while the other four fingers provide support for the thumb (Figure 3-59). Another technique is to grab a muscle and rub or shake it. This is used particularly on the muscles beside the armpit, the arm muscles, the thigh muscles, and the calf muscles (Figure 3-60).

5.   Caressing (Mo)(摸):

Lightly touching the patient's skin can relax the patient and give them a very pleasant feeling. Simply move your hands lightly along the massage pathways. For a more delicate, sensitive feeling, use just your fingertips (Figure 3-61). Follow the simple rules, and massage from the top to the bottom, and from the center to the sides and limbs.

Figure 3-60.

Figure 3-61.

Figure 3-62.

Figure 3-63.

This will help the patient to lead the Qi from the top of the head to the feet and finally to the ground, and it can also help to spread stagnant Qi in the body out to the limbs and finally get rid of it.

6.   Point Striking or Knocking (Dian Da, Qiao)(點打，敲):
Point Striking is tapping or striking specific areas or cavities with the fingertips (Figure 3-62). This stimulates the skin or cavity, and raises stagnant Qi or blood to the surface.

7.   Vibrating (Zhen Zhan)(震顫):
Vibrating is a quick, shaking motion. Normally, this shaking motion is done together with another technique. For example, in Dian Xue massage you will frequently press a cavity with a finger and then shake or vibrate the finger to quickly raise the energy level in the cavity (Figure 3-63). In general and Tui Na massage, you may grab a muscle or tendon and shake it to stimulate it (Figure 3-64).

Figure 3-64.

Figure 3-65.

Figure 3-66.

Figure 3-67.

You may also press with the base of your palm on big muscles such as the trunk and thigh muscles, and then shake them to loosen them up (Figure 3-65).

Vibrating is also commonly done with an up and down motion to stimulate the skin and muscles and increase Qi and blood circulation (Figure 3-66). Qigong masters will often use this technique to lead the Qi into the patient's body for nourishment.

8. Holding (Duan)(端):

Holding is usually used to keep part of the body in a certain position, because different positions will cause the patient's body to respond in different ways. For example, when you are working in the armpit you will want to hold the patient's arm up. Although the muscles in the armpit will be slightly tensed, it will still be much easier for you to reach deeper into the body (Figure 3-67). In Tui Na massage, Holding is used to stabilize the body when you set or relo-

Figure 3-68.   Figure 3-69.

Figure 3-70.

cate bones. While holding part of the body, you may move it in
certain ways to loosen it up. For example, in general massage you
may lift the shoulder and move it to loosen up the shoulder blade
and shoulder (Figure 3-68).

9. Raising or Lifting (Ti)(提):

Raising or Lifting is moving part of the body upward. For
example, when a patient is lying face downward, you may lift up and
lower their waist area to loosen up the muscles there (Figure 3-69).
You may also lift up a patient's head to loosen up the neck muscles
and spine (Figure 3-70), or raise their arms or legs to loosen up the
joints in general massage.

Figure 3-71.

Figure 3-72.

In Qi massage, a Qigong master will place his palms on a cavity and push down gently and firmly, and then, in coordination with his breathing, quickly lift up his palms (Figure 3-71). This sudden change on the surface of the skin will affect the Qi in the patient's body.

10. Pulling (La)(拉):
Pulling is generally applied on the limbs. In general massage, the arms and legs are pulled to straighten out the muscles and tendons (Figure 3-72). In Tui Na massage, Pulling is generally used to set broken bones.

11. Kneading (Nie)(捏):
Kneading is using the thumb and one or more fingers to grab a portion of the patient's body and then either squeeze or rub it. Kneading is different from Grabbing, which is used for larger areas. Kneading is commonly used on the muscles in the back of the neck, the muscles between the neck and the shoulders, the muscles beside the armpit, and on the arms and legs. Very often tendons, such as the ones in the ankles or the back of the knees, are also kneaded in Tui Na massage (Figure 3-73). Sometimes the skin, especially on the back, is kneaded to stimulate the Qi there (Figure 3-74).

12. Supporting (Ding)(頂):
Ding means to support, and it is different from Holding or Raising. Supporting is using part of your body to support part of the patient's body so that you can massage it more easily. For example, you may place the patient's arm on your shoulder and massage the upper arm (Figure 3-75). You may also use your leg to support the patient's leg in order to loosen up the thigh muscles (Figure 3-76).

Figure 3-73.

Figure 3-74.

Figure 3-75.

Figure 3-76.

13. Shaking (Yao)(搖):

Yao means to shake, but it is different from the Vibrating discussed above. The motion of Vibrating is fast and the scale is much smaller, while Shaking is slower and the motion is larger. You may grab a muscle and shake it, such as the muscles between the neck and the shoulder (Figure 3-77), or the muscle on the back of the thigh (Figure 3-78). You may even simply use the thumb or the base of the hand to press down and then shake a muscle to stimulate it (Figure 3-79).

14. Slapping (Pai)(拍):

Slapping is done with either the front or the back of the fingers (Figure 3-80). After slapping to stimulate the Qi in the skin, you may use smooth, gentle pushes to push the stagnant Qi away.

Figure 3-77.

Figure 3-78.

Figure 3-79.

Figure 3-80.

15. Flicking (Tan)(彈):

In Flicking, the thumb holds back the second or the middle finger and then releases it to snap against the skin (Figure 3-81). This stimulates the skin cells and improves Qi circulation in the skin.

16. Swinging (Shuai)(摔):

Swinging is generally used for the limbs. For example, you may gently grab the shoulder or the upper arm and then swing the forearm and the wrist (Figure 3-82). You may also grab the calf and swing the ankle (Figure 3-83). Swinging loosens up a joint so that you can massage it more easily.

Figure 3-81.

Figure 3-82.

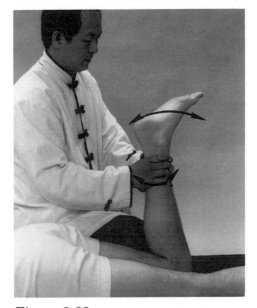

Figure 3-83.

17. Filing (Cuo)(搓):

Filing is rubbing the skin with the side of the palm or the forearm (Figure 3-84). Filing is different from Pushing in that you are rubbing the skin to stimulate it and generate heat. Filing opens the pores and releases the Qi accumulated under the skin.

18. Dividing (Fen)(分):

Dividing is using two forces in opposite directions on a part of the body. For example, you may place both palms on the patient's back and push away from the spine and then let up (Figure 3-85). This stretches the muscles, and when you let up the pressure, the muscles are stimulated. Another example is when you use both thumbs to push the accumulated Qi and blood to the sides of the

Figure 3-84.

Figure 3-85.

Figure 3-86.

Figure 3-87.

forehead and spread them out (Figure 3-86).

Dividing can also be used to stretch the arms and legs. Stretching and then releasing the muscles will stimulate them and help to remove stagnant Qi and blood.

19. Combining (He)(合):

Combining is using two forces to squeeze or bring together parts of the body. For example, you may use both hands to push the muscles or the skin on the sides of the back toward the center (Figure 3-87).

20. Folding (Die)(迭):

Folding is generally used to loosen the joints of the spine or the chest. For example, you may use both hands to fold the entire body

Figure 3-88.

Figure 3-89.

Figure 3-90.

Figure 3-91.

and then release it to loosen it up (Figure 3-88). You may also press both shoulders forward to fold in the chest area, and then release the pressure. This will loosen up the chest (Figure 3-89).

21. Rolling (Gun)(搋):

Rolling is done with the back of the hand near the knuckles. Hold your hand slightly rounded, and keep it relaxed as you roll it back and forth on the area you are treating (Figure 3-90). If you need to apply more power, you may place your other hand on the one you are rolling with and use the power of both arms (Figure 3-91). For rolling on larger areas, such as the back or the thigh, you may use a forearm (Figure 3-92). Rolling massage increases Qi and blood circulation, gets rid of the lactic acid which has accumulated in the

Figure 3-92.

Figure 3-93.

Figure 3-94.

muscles, and also restores feeling in numb areas.

22. Waving (Dou)(抖):

Waving is different from Shaking or Vibrating in that it is a slower, larger motion. To do it, you simply grab one of the patient's limbs and shake it in a large, slow motion (Figure 3-93). Waving loosens the joints, stretches the muscles and tendons, and also increases the Qi and blood circulation.

23. Chopping (Pi)(劈):

Chopping is a strike with the side of the palm (Figure 3-94). It is used when you need increased penetrating power to stimulate the deeper muscles. Chopping is commonly used on the back trunk muscles, the thigh muscles, or sometimes the calf muscles.

Figure 3-95.   Figure 3-96.

Figure 3-97.

24. Carrying On the Back (Bei)(背):

Carrying on the Back is a technique which is used for treating spine problems. As the name indicates, you carry the patient on your back facing either away from you (Figure 3-95) or toward you (Figure 3-96), and swing or shake them gently. This technique stretches the patient's spine and trunk muscles, and releases any tightness in the spine.

25. Piercing (Qia)(掐):

Piercing uses a fingernail (often the thumbnail) to press cavities and stimulate the Qi circulation (Figure 3-97). Of course, the fingernail should not break the skin. Piercing is sometimes used by physicians who do not have acupuncture needles. Piercing is commonly

Figure 3-98.

Figure 3-99.

used in both Tui Na and Dian Xue massage. Pressing in with a fingernail can quickly stimulate a cavity, so Piercing is commonly used to revive people who have fainted, or to quickly make the body more Yang, for example when a patient has a cold.

26. Pointing (Dian)(點):

Pointing uses a finger (usually the thumb, or the index or middle finger), or two fingers (usually the index and middle fingers) to press heavily on a cavity (Figure 3-98). Pointing is different from Pressing, which was discussed previously. The area covered with Pressing can be large or small, however, Pointing covers a much smaller area, and its power is more penetrating. Sometimes the elbow is used when you need more power to penetrate to a cavity which is covered by a thick layer of muscle, such as in the thigh (Figure 3-99). The Pointing technique is sometimes used when acupuncture needles are not available. Pointing is mainly used for Tui Na and Dian Xue massage.

27. Transporting (Yun)(運):

Transporting uses the fingers to rub repeatedly in a straight line or circle until the skin is warm (Figure 3-100). This technique is usually applied on small children. However, it is sometimes used for adults in massaging the chest, abdomen, and face. When you are doing the Transporting technique, your fingers should lightly touch the skin as they rub with a fairly fast motion.

28. Quick Pull (Che)(扯):

The Quick Pull technique is commonly used to loosen up joints in the arms and legs. To do this technique, hold a finger, a wrist, or ankle and move it around to loosen it up, and then give it a quick

Figure 3-100.

Figure 3-101.

Figure 3-102.

pull (Figure 3-101). This technique is different from the Pulling technique described in #10. While #10 pulls with a steady, firm power, Quick Pull uses a quick jerk. Quick Pull is commonly used on people who are strong but have very tense joints.

29. Extending (Shen)(伸):

Extending is used to straighten a bent limb. Pain usually causes muscles and tendons to contract, which keeps the arm or leg in a bent position. Extending is needed to straighten the limb. To use Extending, hold the limb on both sides of the constricted joint and pull in both directions with a firm and steady power (Figure 3-102). Do not use violent power, because that will only cause more tension.

30. Bending (Qu)(曲):

Bending is the reverse of Extending. When a patient's arm or leg is straight and cannot be bent because of stiffness or numbness, you

Figure 3-103.

Figure 3-104.

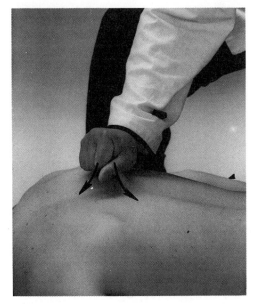

Figure 3-105.

want to bend it to loosen up the joints. Hold the limb on both sides of the joint and bend it with steady, firm power (Figure 3-103). Normally, Bending and Extending are repeated until the joint is completely loose.

31. Striking (Da)(打):

Striking uses the fists to strike an area (Figure 3-104). You need to carefully gauge the power, since too much force will cause bruises or other injuries, while too little force will not be effective. You want to stimulate the nervous system and Qi without causing any damage. Striking is used to quickly stimulate an area in the same way that, when your leg has fallen asleep, you punch it to restore feeling.

32. Shifting, Slipping (Nuo)(挪):

To do Shifting, grab a piece of skin with one or both hands, and either shake it or let it slip out of your hand (Figure 3-105). Shifting

Figure 3-107.

Figure 3-106.

is used to stimulate the skin, but be careful when you grab not to damage the skin. Shifting is commonly used on the back.

33. Reining (Le)(勒):

Reining is commonly used to stretch the muscles or tendons on the joints of the fingers or toes. To do Reining, hold the patient's wrist or ankle with one hand, and hold the finger or toe you are treating with the thumb and index finger of your other hand. Pull the finger, and then let it quickly slip out of your grip (Figure 3-106). Reining is slightly different from Pulling, in which you hold the patient's limb steadily, without letting it slide out of your grip.

34. Uprooting (Ba)(拔):

In Uprooting, you grab a piece of skin, muscle, or tendon and pull it away from the body (Figure 3-107). Uprooting is commonly used to stimulate the skin or the muscles located under the armpit, between the neck and the shoulder, elbows, or the hips.

35. Squeezing (Ji)(擠):

Squeezing is commonly done with the fingers or palms. The fingers are used on smaller areas of skin, such as on the forehead or the smaller joints such as the spinal joints in the neck (Figure 3-108). The palms are used to squeeze the big muscles in the arms and legs (Figure 3-109).

36. Twisting (Ban)(扳):

Twisting is commonly used for the neck. Hold the back of the head and the chin, and give a quick twist to the side with both hands (Figure 3-110). Twisting is used to loosen the neck joints and also stretch the neck muscles and tendons.

Figure 3-108.

Figure 3-109.

Figure 3-110.

Figure 3-111.

37. Threshing (Dao)(搗):

Threshing is commonly used to stimulate a cavity or a small, specific area with a continuous up and down or sideways movement. Threshing uses the index finger, supported by the thumb and middle finger (Figure 3-111), or a joint of the index finger (Figure 3-112). Press in on the cavity or area and move up and down or sideways with a steady speed until the area is sufficiently stimulated.

Figure 3-112.

Figure 3-113.

Figure 3-114.

38. Pecking (Zhuo)(啄):

Pecking uses the fingertips formed into a beak to stimulate the skin (Figure 3-113). Pecking is different from the Tapping technique described earlier in that Pecking focuses on a smaller area, while Tapping covers a wider area.

39. Swaying (Huang)(晃):

With the Swaying technique you place both hands on the patient's body and move the skin to and fro with a very slow motion (Figure 3-114). Swaying is used to relax the patient physically and mentally. Be sure not to rub the skin, just move it back and forth.

Figure 3-115.

Figure 3-116.

Figure 3-117.

Figure 3-118.

40. Rotating (Xuan)(旋):

Rotating is commonly used for joints in the limbs. Hold the limb on both sides of the joint and twist (Figure 3-115) or rotate the joint (Figure 3-116). Twisting the limb will stretch the muscles, while rotating the joint will loosen the joint.

41. Combing (Shu)(梳):

This technique uses the fingers or fingertips to comb along the ribs from the center of the body to the sides (Figure 3-117). Combing is one of the main techniques for leading Qi from the center of the body to the sides.

42. Scratching (Sao)(搔):

Scratching, which is done just as the name indicates, is used on specific areas such as the head (Figure 3-118). This technique is

Figure 3-119.   Figure 3-120.

used to stimulate an area, or to bring Qi to it. A light scratch will soothe, while a heavier scratch will stimulate.

43. Reeling (Chan)(纏):
Reeling uses the middle section of the fingers and palms to rub in a circular motion along a straight line (Figure 3-119). Reeling can be used on most of the body, such as the back, the chest, or the limbs.

44. Scraping (Gua)(刮):
Scraping uses the fingernails or the knuckles to scrape the skin (Figure 3-120). This technique is commonly used in Tui Na along the Qi channels or on areas corresponding to specific internal organs to regulate the Qi there.

45. Jabbing (Lu)(戮):
Jabbing uses a fingertip to press straight downward on a cavity to stimulate it (Figure 3-121). Usually the tip of the index or middle finger is used. Jabbing is a common technique in Dian Xue Massage. Jabbing is sometimes considered to be part of the Pointing technique; the main difference is that Jabbing is always used straight downward.

46. Pounding (Guan)(貫):
Pounding is a technique for indirectly applying the force of a fist strike. Usually, one hand is placed on the area being treated, and it is struck with the other fist. This technique is usually used on the top of the head (Figure 3-122) or the bottom of the feet (Figure 3-123), and with only mild power.

47. Cascading (Qie)(切):
Cascading uses the fingernails to slowly stimulate many spots on an area of the body in a special order (Figures 3-124 and 3-125). Each finger stimulates a point in immediate succession, like a water-

Figure 3-121.

Figure 3-122.

Figure 3-123.

Figure 3-124.

fall flowing through rocks. This strongly stimulates the skin, and leads Qi from under the skin to the surface.

48. Wiping (Cha)(擦):
Wiping uses the fingers or palm to gently wipe or brush to and fro on the area being massaged (Figure 3-126). Wiping is an easy way to stimulate the skin cells. It is commonly used to strengthen deficient Guardian Qi.

49. Dredging (Tao)(掏):
Dredging uses the thumb or the last section of one or more fingers to press on a cavity and then drag outward (Figure 3-127). Dredging is commonly used in Tui Na and Dian Xue massage. When using Dredging, be careful not to break the skin.

Figure 3-125.

Figure 3-126.

Figure 3-127.

Figure 3-128.

50. Cupping (Kou)(叩):

To use Cupping, cup your hand with all the fingers touching, and hit the area you are treating (Figure 3-128). Cupping can stimulate the skin efficiently without injuring it.

These are only some of the many techniques which have been used by masseurs around the world. This section is meant only to offer a guideline and some examples to help you understand the massage techniques. As long as you remember the purpose of massage and the theory behind it, you should be able to apply the different techniques skillfully.

3-4. The Keys to Successful Massage

The best way to master massage is to learn the theory and then apply it in practice. As a beginner, the best way to gain massage experience is to practice on yourself. This will let you feel the power, understand how the body responds, and see the results. The next step is to catch every opportunity to massage people who are also interested in massaging you. The mutual exchange of experiences and ideas will help you to grasp the key points very easily.

To reach a higher level of training, it is necessary to practice Qigong. Qigong emphasizes the methods of regulating the body, breathing, mind, Qi, and spirit. All of these are required to reach a profound level of understanding in massage. Next, let us discuss these requirements.

1. Regulating the Body:

We have mentioned earlier how important it is to help your patients regulate their bodies until they are relaxed, centered, and balanced. However, you must also do the same for yourself. Whether you are massaging yourself or someone else, the first thing you need to do is to relax your body and to find the most comfortable position. This will help you to find your mental center and balance, which is an absolute necessity for determining what your patient needs and evaluating the results of your massage. For example, if you are tense and nervous, then your patient will also be tense, and your massage will be ineffective.

2. Regulating the Breathing:

When you massage yourself or someone else, you should remember that massage is part of Chinese Qigong, and, in many cases, it is even harder to practice than Qigong. When you are massaging someone, you are not just dealing with yourself, but with another person's physical and Qi bodies. You need to be able to reach the patient's mind and feel their feelings, and become one with them, not just in your mind, but in actuality.

In Qigong, breathing is the key strategy when you use your mind to direct the Qi. The goal of Qigong practice is to unite your body, breathing, and mind, which causes your Qi body to be smoothly and harmoniously distributed in your physical body. Breathing strategy also plays a crucial role in Qigong massage. For example, when the patient is exhaling, they are instinctively leading Qi to the surface of the skin, and when they are inhaling, they are leading it deep into the body. If you coordinate your power with the patient's breathing, your massage can reach deep into their body. For example, in Dian Xue massage, your power can penetrate much more deeply if you apply it when the patient is inhaling.

The other side of the coin is your breathing when you are giving a massage. When you exhale, you are leading Qi to your extremities much more strongly than when you inhale. For example, when you use Dian Xue massage, if you wish to use your Qi to nourish the patient's Qi, you must press when you are exhaling to be effective. Naturally, if you wish to remove excess Qi from the patient, you should do it as you are inhaling. You can see that it is not just your mind which builds the bridge between you and your patient, but also your breathing.

3. Regulating the Mind:

The mind is the general in charge of the entire massage. It is the mind which coordinates every aspects of what is happening. In Qigong massage, when your mind is in a meditative state your massage will be much more coordinated, and your understanding of the process will be much deeper. Therefore, to massage effectively your mind must be concentrated, and it must be able to reach the patient's mind.

4. Regulating the Qi:

In order to use massage to regulate the patient's Qi, you must first regulate your own Qi. If your Qi circulation is abnormal and unbalanced, how can you possibly regulate the patient's Qi? If you try to help someone regulate their Qi, but your own Qi is unhealthy, you will not be able to judge the situation clearly, and you will only make things worse. Furthermore, sometimes the patient's excess Qi will overflow into your own body. If you do not know how to regulate this problem, it can bring you harm. This is the reason why people practicing Qigong massage should also be Qigong practitioners.

5. Regulating the Shen (spirit):

The spirit is a product of the mind, your willingness to share, your concern, and your sincerity. If you have a good level of Qi communication with your patient, you can also start increasing the degree of spiritual communication. This will act as a catalyst, and enhance the effectiveness of your treatment. The greatest source of healing is within the patient. If you raise their spirit you increase their confidence in the healing, and their Qi can be led more effectively and efficiently. This is the key to an effective spiritual healing.

These training concepts will give you an idea of how to reach the higher levels of massage. However, actually achieving them may take a very long time. As long as you remember these five criteria of massage and keep working toward them, the more experience you accumulate, the better you will become. These requirements are usually not so critical in general or relaxation massage. However, when you enter into Tui Na, Dian Xue, and Qi massage, these requirements become the keys to success.

Reference

(*1). "The Body Electric" by Robert O. Becker, M.D. and Gary Selden, Quill, William Morrow, New York, 1985.

PART TWO

GENERAL MASSAGE

Chapter 4
General Concepts

4-1. Introduction

One of the more enjoyable experiences in life is to get a general massage to help you relax and recover from fatigue. Unlike Tui Na or Dian Xue massage, which are designed to heal, general massage can help you to relax mentally and spiritually, while physically it can help to disperse stagnant Qi and blood, speeding recovery from fatigue. This kind of massage is especially beneficial for older people, because it helps maintain the smooth circulation of Qi and blood, consequently slowing down the aging process. Normally, the blood and Qi circulation gradually become sluggish as we get older.

The luxury of general massage is known in almost every culture, so there are many variations in theory and techniques. Even in China there are countless styles of general massage for relaxation. However, they all share the same basic theory. I believe that as long as you have mastered the theory and the techniques of one style, it will be easy for you to grasp the key to any other style. Remember, when you learn something, **DON'T LEARN MANY THINGS SUPERFICIALLY. INSTEAD, LEARN A FEW THINGS DEEPLY.** When you learn deeply, you will grasp the theory, which is the root. If your knowledge is wide and shallow, you have only learned about the branches.

In order to master general massage, you must learn and ponder the theory, study the techniques, and gain a lot of experience. The more you think and ponder, the more deeply you will understand. The more you practice, the greater your skill will be. The more experience you accumulate, the wider your knowledge will be. These three things are the keys to success. Keep on the path, and be humble, persevering, and patient. One day you will discover that the fruits of the seed you have planted are bigger and sweeter than anyone else's.

Most people who learn massage start with general massage, because you do not need a deep understanding of the Qi circulation system or a high degree of skill. General massage teaches you the structure of the body and lets you feel the pattern of the Qi flow in the energy body. These understandings are crucial if you wish to learn Tui Na and Dian Xue massage.

General massage includes self-massage and massage with a partner. From the point of view of training, self-massage starts you on the path to mastering the skills of massage and building up a store of experience. It is therefore desirable to start with self-massage.

In our discussion, however, we will start with massage with a partner. It is important for the beginner to have a good understanding of the structure of the body as well as an overview of the complete massage procedure. However, this is difficult to learn in self massage, since it is difficult to reach many parts of your own body, such as your back and hips.

In this chapter we will first review the purposes of general massage, then its theory, and finally its procedures and rules. In Chapter 5 we will discuss the techniques used in massaging the various parts of your partner's body. Before we introduce the techniques for each part of the body, we will review the structure of our physical and Qi bodies. We will focus especially on the networks of the nervous system and the Qi, blood, and lymph circulatory systems, as well as the gates or junctions. Finally, in Chapter 6 we will discuss self-massage. Since we have already discussed the basic theory and rules, we will not repeat them there. Self-massage will be divided into three sections: external self-massage, internal organ self-massage by hand, and finally, internal organ self-massage through movement.

4-2. Purposes of General Massage

Before you practice general massage, you should first ponder several questions: 1. Why do you want to practice general massage, and what are your goals? 2. How do you intend to reach these goals? 3. What are the theories behind general massage? The first question shows you your motivation and also your target. Without knowing the answer to this question, your mind will be uncertain and confused. The second and third questions actually cannot be separated. Theory is the Yin side of practice, and it gives you the structured knowledge that lies behind the techniques. You need to have a profound understanding of the theory before you can choose the appropriate methods and techniques to reach your goals. These methods and techniques are the "how, " which is the Yang, the manifestation of Yin.

In this and the following sections we will discuss the "why" and "what" of general massage. After explaining the theory, we will list a few general rules drawn from the theoretical analysis. After we have built this theoretical foundation, we will discuss the "how" in the following chapters.

Although we have already discussed the purposes of general massage in an earlier section, we would like to summarize them again here to develop the connection with the subjects that follow.

A. Releasing Mental Tension:

Mental tension comes from thinking (i.e., from your mind). According to Chinese Qigong, the mind is the "general" of your Qigong training, since it controls your entire being including both your Qi and physical bodies. Whenever your peace of mind is disturbed, the Qi circulation in your body will be immediately affected. For example, if your mind is disturbed by sadness, your Qi will be led inward to be stored in your bone marrow. When this happens you will feel cold, because the Qi in the muscles and skin is deficient (i.e., the Guardian Qi is condensed and weak). Conversely, if your mind is excited from happiness, there will be an excess of Qi in the muscles and skin, and you will feel hot (i.e., the Guardian Qi is expanding and strong). Whenever there is a deficiency of Qi (Yin) or an excess (Yang), the physical body will react accordingly, since its condition is decided by the Qi. Whenever the Qi supply to the physical body is abnormal (either Yin or Yang), the physical body will be tense, and this tension will cause the circulation of the Qi and blood to be sluggish.

Therefore, the first goal of general massage is to relieve mental tension. This restores normal Qi circulation, and insures that the cells of the physical body receive the proper amount of Qi nourishment. The greatest benefit of releasing mental tension is the relief from stress and depression, which brings the happiness back into your life.

B. Removing Stagnant Qi and Blood:

Stagnant Qi and blood can have many causes such as mental stress and tension, improper lifestyle, fatigue, aging, and sickness.

Improper lifestyle includes the food you eat, the air you breathe, the time you get up and how long you sleep. In Chinese Qigong, food and air are the post-birth essences which can be converted into Qi. If you eat improper food and breathe unclean air, your body will produce poor quality Qi. Furthermore, some of the undesirable materials can remain in your body. For example, undigested fat can be stored in the body. We know that fat can cause sluggish circulation of Qi and blood. Our Qi circulation can also be affected by the time of day (i.e., by the sun's Qi). Therefore, working the night shift may disturb your Qi. Another example is that you usually need at least seven to eight hours of sleep to replenish the energy of your brain and body. If you do not get enough sleep, your Qi circulation can be affected and also the quality of your blood cells may be poor.

Another common cause of sluggish Qi and blood circulation is overwork and fatigue. Overwork causes your body to generate more waste (such as lactic acid) than the blood can remove. When the acid accumulates in the muscles, you feel tired, and your body becomes even more tense, which further affects the Qi circulation. One of the most effective methods of recovering from fatigue, other than rest, is general massage.

Aging is the next cause of stagnant Qi and blood circulation. As you get older, especially after thirty when the body stops producing growth hormones, your blood and muscle cells start to age. The blood cells are not as fresh and the Qi is not as abundant as when you were young. When this happens, the circulation of Qi and blood becomes sluggish. General massage will maintain and improve the circulation.

Finally, Qi and blood circulation can also be affected by illness. We will discuss this further in the sections on Tui Na and Dian Xue massage.

C. Maintaining a Healthy Nervous System:

When the circulation of Qi and blood is smooth and healthy, it will provide proper nourishment to the entire body including the nervous system. Nerves connect the brain to the entire body, and enable the brain to govern it, and they also enable the body to respond to the brain. Without a good communication system, you will lose the war against sickness and aging. General massage helps the nervous system to function properly by insuring that it receives the proper amount of Qi nourishment.

D. Increasing Hormone Production and Strengthening the Immune System:

The production of hormones and the condition of the lymphatic system are closely related to the immune system. Although we still do not understand exactly how the hormones work, we do know that they provide significant benefits. Only recently it was reported that the growth hormone can significantly extend the life span.

The endocrine and lymphatics systems are like factories. If we want to maintain or even increase production, we have to consider how to increase the energy supply to them. The lymphatic system is an important part of our body's defense against bacteria. I would like to point out again that the Qi circulatory system (the Yin system) is the root of all other circulatory systems.

E. For Enjoyment:

The fact that it is so enjoyable is probably the main reason that most people are drawn to general massage. Not only does it help you to calm your mind and find peace, it can also bring you to a stage of deep relaxation and a feeling of complete comfort. In the beginning, it is difficult to bring your partner to this state. However, as your understanding of Qigong deepens, and as you gain experience, you will find that it happens more and more easily.

In conclusion, general massage has three areas of benefit: mental, Qi, and physical. The mental area is related to the mind, the Qi area to the inner energy which is the root of life, and the physical area is the body which manifests life. Although we discuss these three areas independently, they are closely related and cannot be separated. To maintain and improve your health, you need to be concerned with all three of them.

4-3. Theory of General Massage

We have explained in Part One that each category of massage has different purposes, and so each category has its own unique theory and somewhat different ways of reaching its goals. In general massage, to obtain the maximum result you need to massage the mental body first, then the physical body, and finally the Qi body. No matter how hard you try to massage someone, or how strong your Qi is, if their mind is not calm and peaceful, you are wasting your time. However, when your partner can mentally coordinate with your massage, they will be able to relax deep inside and help you work. When the body is relaxed, the Qi can circulate more smoothly, and it can be led more easily. You have to massage your partner's mind before you massage the physical body. You can see that when you massage, you are massaging three different bodies, yet you must treat them as one. They are mutually related and cannot be separated.

1. Massaging the Mental Body:

When you are massaging someone, your first concern is how to gain their whole-hearted mental and physical cooperation. Since the main purpose of massage is to improve the Qi and blood circulation, if your partner's mind remains tense, their physical body will also be tense and their Qi circulation stagnant. In addition, tense muscles may cause the pulse to speed up, and may even raise their blood pressure. Remember: **IN A GOOD MASSAGE, THE PERSON BEING MASSAGED SHOULD BE IN A SEMI-HYPNOTIC, RELAXED, MEDITATIVE STATE.** When this happens, the heart beat slows down and the mind is very peaceful. This does not mean that the person being massaged should be asleep. If you want to efficiently improve their Qi and blood circulation, you need their whole-hearted cooperation. Remember, **IT IS THE YI WHICH LEADS THE QI.** When your partner's Yi (mind) is with your massage, they can regulate their Qi more efficiently, and your massage can be most effective. However, if your partner falls asleep, then the massage will not be as successful.

Furthermore, when you massage someone, you want your massage to reach well past their skin and muscles and deep into their body, as deep as the internal organs and bone marrow. However, when people give general massages they frequently cannot get their power to penetrate deeply enough. The cause of the problem is often with the person being massaged. They must be calm, they must be relaxed and balanced both mentally and physically, and most important of all, they must use their own meditative mind to regulate the Qi and blood circulation.

When you do have the cooperation of your massage partner, your Qi will unite with their Qi, your mind will unite with their mind, and both of you will enjoy the massage. As you can see, in general massage, your first task is to massage your partner's mind and spirit before you start on the physical massage.

2. Massaging the Physical Body:

The main purpose of physical massage is to stimulate the cells of the body, enhancing Qi and blood circulation and removing Qi and blood stagnation. Massaging the physical body includes massage of the nerve endings (i.e., the skin), the sensory organs (ears, eyes, nose, and mouth), the fasciae and muscles, the joints including the spine, the internal organs, and the bone marrow.

A. Massaging the Nerve Endings:

When you massage the nerve endings, you are actually also massaging the endings of the Qi channels in the skin. The nervous system communicates feelings and sensations to your brain, and your brain directs the Qi. Since the nervous system and the Qi system are so closely related, it is not surprising that massage techniques used on the skin can adjust both systems.

Massaging the nerve endings in the skin enables you to maintain or even improve the connection between them and the brain. Usually, when you touch the skin in the proper way, you can relax the entire part of the nervous system which is related to that area of the skin. This is why we can use touch to express our emotions so well and cause such varied sensations in our partners. So much love can be communicated through the sense of touch.

There are three ways to physically massaging the skin. The first way is by using a gentle touch along the massage pathways (i.e., from the top to the bottom and from the center to the sides). This kind of massage can relax your partner and also lead them into a meditative state. Usually, this kind of skin massage is done at the very beginning of the massage.

The second way of massaging the skin is by slapping, grabbing and shaking, or even by whipping the body with the appropriate equipment. This type of massage causes some degree of pain, but it strongly stimulates the nerve endings and brings Qi and blood hidden deeply in or under the muscles to the surface of the skin allowing it to disperse. In Greece, this type of massage is done by gently hitting the skin with branches. This kind of skin massage is done near the end of the massage, when the Qi and blood accumulated deep within the body have already been loosened up. Slapping or gently whipping the skin will then lead the Qi and blood to the surface of the skin where it can be spread out.

The third way of massaging the skin is to rub it with the hands to generate heat, which leads the accumulated Qi and blood to the skin and spreads it out.

B. Massaging the Sensory Organs:

In addition to massaging the skin, which is the sensory organ of touch, we must also massage the other sensory organs: the eyes, ears, nose, and mouth. In Chinese medicine, the areas near these organs are considered to be the endings of the Qi channels. As you get older, the Qi circulation to these organs gets weaker, and they don't function as well. The degeneration of vision and hearing are common occurences in old age. Because of this, general massage places great emphasis on massaging the sensory organs.

Massaging around the sensory organs will gently stimulate the nervous system to lead Qi and blood to them. In fact, many people have had their vision and hearing improved through massage after years of deterioration.

C. Massaging the Muscles and Fasciae:

Massaging the muscles and fasciae is probably the most important aspect of general massage for fatigue, although, of course, it can also greatly relax you even when you are not fatigued. When you are fatigued, an excessive amount of lactic acid has accumulated in the muscles. This causes muscle pain and the accumulation of Qi and blood.

When you massage the muscles, you are also massaging the fasciae between the skin and the muscles, and between the layers of muscle. The fat which is stored in the fascia hinders the Qi and blood circulation. General massage can remove much of this stored fat.

When you massage the muscles and fasciae, you stimulate them and increase the circulation of Qi and blood. This removes the lactic acid and spreads it out so that it can be removed from your system. Since most of the Qi channels are within the muscles, this will also restore smooth Qi circulation, which is one of the best ways of retarding the aging process.

D. Massaging the Spine:

The spine consists of seven cervical vertebrae in the neck, twelve thoracic vertebrae in the back, five lumber vertebrae in the waist, as well as the sacrum and tailbone. Nerves branch out from the spinal cord to the limbs and the internal organs. Any problem with the spinal cord interferes with the brain's ability to sense and govern the body.

Inside the spinal column is a Qi vessel (the Thrusting Vessel) which connects the brain to the Huiyin cavity and communicates with the other two main vessels (the Conception and Governing Vessels). These three vessels are the most important ones in the body, and they are intimately related to your health and longevity. Whenever the Qi level in these three vessels is low, the whole body receives insufficient Qi nourishment, and consequently, the physical body (including the nervous system) cannot function normally.

In order to keep enough Qi coming into the central nervous system, the spine must be loose, and any accumulated Qi or blood must be removed. Since the trunk muscles around the spine have a very great influence on the condition of the spine, massaging the trunk muscles is a very important part of spine massage.

E. Massaging the Joints:

This refers to the joints in the arms and legs. We know that in the area of the joints are gates which allow the exchange of Qi between the body and the environment. In addition, around the joints are areas where we can access the main nerves and arteries. And, of course, the joints allow us to move our limbs freely. Whenever there is any stagnation of Qi or blood in the joints, or any physical defect such as arthritis, we suffer pain and our mobility is limited. Injuries and aging affect the joints much more than the shafts of the bones. Therefore, general massage places great emphasis on keeping the joints healthy and functioning properly.

F. Massaging the Internal Organs:

The internal organs can be massaged with the hands and also with movement. While another person can use the first method on you, you may use either one on yourself.

When you massage by hand, you place your hands on the skin above the organ, and use gentle rubbing movements in specific patterns to loosen the muscles around the organ. The gentle movements of your hands generate Qi under the skin. This Qi follows the movement of the hands, and therefore can be directed into the organ. Naturally, if the person being massaged uses their mind to relax the muscles and lead the Qi, the results will be significantly greater.

Massage by movement uses mainly the trunk muscles and the up and down movement of the diaphragm (from deep breathing) to massage the internal organs. Muscles in the torso wrap around the internal organs. When these muscles are tense, the Qi and blood circulation around the internal organs will be stagnant. Therefore, the first steps of self-massage of the internal organs with movement are learning how to loosen up the trunk muscles, and then using movements of the trunk muscles to massage the internal organs. You also need to learn how to breathe deeply to move the diaphragm smoothly, slowly, and gently while keeping it relaxed. This massages the organs under the diaphragm.

In Qigong, it is desirable to learn how to control the muscles in the abdominal area so that you can move the abdomen in and out. This will enhance the effectiveness of the internal organ massage.

G. Massaging the Bone Marrow:

Massaging the bone marrow is one of the most difficult parts of general massage. The main purpose of bone marrow massage is to lead Qi to the marrow to maintain the normal production of healthy blood cells. In Chinese Qigong, one of the most effective ways of leading Qi to the marrow is through correct breathing techniques and certain methods of meditation. These are discussed in the YMAA book "Muscle/Tendon Changing and Marrow/Brain Washing Chi Kung."

Because the theory is difficult to understand, most practitioners of Qigong massage have ignored marrow massage. I would like to introduce several possible massage techniques which may stimulate the Qi circulation in the marrow.

The first technique is stimulating the bones in the area of the joints, where the bone is most exposed and closest to the skin. The

Figure 4-1.

Figure 4-2. Bone breathing through muscle stimulation.

shaft of the bone is protected by the muscles and difficult to reach. To stimulate the bone at the joint, press the bone with your fingernails and circle your fingers (Figure 4-1). Move the skin with your nails so that you do not scrape the skin. This will cause a slight amount of pain, and in some areas, such as the knees, it will cause an exciting, stimulating sensation deep within the body. You may also use your teeth to stimulate the bones at the joints or at places which do not have a thick layer of muscle over them, such as the shin. Go very carefully. Do not cause too much pain, and do not cause any bruising, because that would make the entire body more tense, and you will not be able to accomplish your goal.

In the areas which are protected by a thick layer of muscle, you can increase the exchange of Qi by stimulating the muscles so that Qi is led from the marrow to the skin (Figure 4-2). When this happens, the bone draws fresh Qi from around the joint. The easiest way to do this is to use a whip made of wire or a bar (Figure 4-3) to gently hit the muscles until they get warm.

3. Massaging the Qi Body:

First, I would like to point out that massaging the Qi body is different from Qi massage, which we will discuss in the second volume of this book. When you massage the Qi body, you use both physical techniques and Qi correspondence to regulate your partner's Qi. However, in Qi massage, you cause your Qi to correspond with your partner's Qi so that you can regulate and rebalance it. Massaging the Qi body smoothes the Qi circulation for relaxation and health,

Figure 4-3. Wire whip.

while Qi massage is used to correct abnormal Qi circulation which was caused by illness or injury.

Before we discuss massaging the Qi body, I would like to remind you of a very important point we made in the first part of this book. According to both Chinese and Western medicine, every blood cell must have Qi or bioelectricity to stay alive. Furthermore, each blood cell functions like a battery, and stores and releases Qi as needed. Because of this, Qi and blood cannot be completely separated, and when you discuss either one of them, the other one is usually also involved to some degree.

In addition to the blood circulatory system, there are twelve primary channels which also circulate Qi in the body. Most of the course of each channel lies within muscle, so when you tense your muscles you are limiting the Qi circulation to the organs (which are connected to these channels), and they may not receive the proper amount of Qi nourishment. This is why keeping your body relaxed is one of the main keys to health.

Next, we will discuss the theory of how to massage the Qi body.

A. Massaging the Qi Endings:

Massaging the Qi endings cannot be separated from massaging the nerve endings. The reason for this is quite simple. Since Qi is necessary for keeping the nerve fibers alive, small Qi channels supply the nerves, and the endings of these tiny Qi channels are located near the endings of the nerves.

While the skin separates the insides of our bodies from the outside environment, the skin has thousands of pores, capillaries, nerve endings, and small Qi channels through which Qi and air pass in and out. According to Chinese medicine, all of the Qi channel endings in our skin are related to our internal organs. Stimulating the skin can maintain the exchange of air and Qi between our insides and the world outside, and can also stimulate our internal organs.

To massage the Qi endings in the skin, simply touch your partner lightly and move your hands along the massage paths (which are also the routes of the Qi channels and nerves). Move from the top to the bottom, and from the center to the sides. This allows several things to take place. If your Qi is in correspondence with your partner's, they will be able to use their own mind to lead their Qi in synchronization with your movements to smooth their own Qi. This skin-to-skin contact also allows the Qi to pass between you and your partner so that you can nourish each other. Mutual Qi nourishment is one of the methods which Chinese Qigong uses to balance irregular Qi conditions. For example, when you are sad, the Qi in your body is Yin and weak. If a friend holds your hands or hugs you, you immediately receive Qi nourishment from them. This allows you to smooth out your Qi, and helps them to relax. Touching is a natural, instinctive method of Qigong healing.

B. Massaging the Qi Gates:

In general massage, you want to lead the excess Qi out of your partner's body to release the tension. In order to do this, you must know all of the Qi gates and junctions. This includes the gates between the body and the surrounding environment, and also the gates and junctions within the body. Stimulating the gates in sequence along the channels will lead the excess Qi to the limbs and finally release it from the body.

C. Massaging the Endocrine Glands:

An important purpose of general massage is increasing the production of hormones and strengthening the immune system. The production of hormones can be increased in two places in men and in one place in women. In men, this can be done in the adrenal glands, which are on top of the kidneys, and in the testicles. In women, only the adrenal glands can be easily reached. Massaging the muscles around the kidneys and testicles will lead Qi to them and increase hormone production, and will also maintain smooth Qi circulation around them.

4-4. Rules of General Massage

Now that you have a grasp of the theory, you probably already have an idea of what procedure you should follow. In this subsection, I would like to summarize the procedures of general massage, as well as the pathways you should follow, and also to discuss how much power you should use.

1. Procedures:

When you massage, unless you are only massaging a portion of the body, you should follow the standard procedures which tell you where you should start, and where you should end. Following the correct procedures will make the massage more effective and more enjoyable.

A. Mental Massage:

In order to achieve maximum effectiveness, and reach the deepest places in the body, your partner should be in a semi-hypnotic, meditative state. This lets them relax their body as much as possible, which allows the power of the massage to penetrate as deeply as possible. When their mind is calm, they are also able to regulate their own Qi and physical body. Therefore, before the physical massage, you should massage your partner's mental body and help them to enter a deep meditative state.

B. Head and Neck:

In physical massage, it is important to start from the head, because this is where a person's "headquarters" is. Within the head is the brain, which controls the entire body through the nervous system. If the head is tense, the mind will also be tense, as well as the rest of the body.

The neck is the passageway of the Qi and blood. Whenever the neck is tense, the Qi and blood circulation will be stagnant, and the brain will not receive proper nourishment. The best way to remove the excess Qi and blood which has accumulated in the head, as well as to bring in plenty of nourishment, is to relax the neck and keep all of the Qi and blood vessels open.

C. Back:

The next place to massage is the back. The spine is the central supply line of Qi, with the Governing Vessel running up the back of it. The Governing Vessel controls the six primary Yang Qi channels in the body. In addition, in the center of the spine is the Thrusting Vessel, through which the Qi communicates between the lower part of the body and the brain. Furthermore, the spinal cord is a major part of the central nervous system, and all of the peripheral nervous system branches out from it. You can see that the spine is the connection between the brain and the entire body. Whenever there is any problem in the spine, there will be a malfunction in the related portion of the body. This is why loosening up the spine and improving the Qi circulation there is a crucial part of general massage.

After loosening up the spine, the next task is leading the accumulated Qi or blood away from the spine. This Qi and blood, which have accumulated deep inside the joints of the spine, are the main cause of problems with the nervous system. The Qi and blood must be brought up to the skin and spread out to the sides and downward.

D. Back of the Legs:

Excess Qi is released out of the body at the ends of the limbs. The Qi which you have released from the back should be brought out to the limbs. You normally do the legs next, because the Qi channels in the legs are more open than those in the arms. In addition, it is easier to lead the Qi downward than to the sides. Therefore, the next step is to lead the Qi to the bottom of the feet.

E. Back of the Arms:

After you have massaged the legs and feet, you massage the arms to smooth out the Qi flow and lead any excess Qi away from the body. Leading Qi to the arms is one of the most effective ways of releasing excess Qi in the head, simply because the arms are closer to the head than are the legs.

F. Chest and Abdomen:

After you have completed the massage of the back, have your partner turn face upward.

Before you start massaging the chest and abdomen, you need to help your partner regain a meditative state, which was probably disturbed when they turned over. Spend a short time massaging their head to assist them in regaining a meditative state.

The chest and abdomen, which contain most of the internal organs, are the third most important area in general massage. Your goal in massaging this area is to loosen up and relax the muscles in the front of the body, and also to improve the Qi circulation in the internal organs. Your health this determined, in great part, by the condition of your internal organs. Bringing up the Qi and blood which have accumulated in and around the internal organs improves the Qi circulation and helps keep the organs healthy.

G. Front of the Legs:

After you have loosened up the chest and abdomen and brought the accumulated Qi and blood up to the surface, lead the Qi and blood down the legs to the bottom of the feet. Follow the same theory that you used on the back of the legs.

H. Front of the Arms:

Finally, massage the arms and lead the Qi from the head and the front of the body to the arms and get rid of it.

This suggested massage procedure for the entire body is drawn from the theoretical understanding of the Qi and the physical bodies. If you do not have time to massage the entire body, still follow the same sequence with the parts that you do massage. For example, when you massage the head to relieve a headache, also massage the back and arms in order to lead the Qi downward and sideways. If you fail to do this, the Qi and blood will remain in the head. Similarly, when you massage the back to relieve a backache, also massage the legs to lead the Qi further downward.

2. Pathways:

One of the most important factors in successful Qigong massage is following the correct pathways. This is especially true in Tui Na, Dian Xue, and Qi massage. In this section we will discuss only the pathways used in general massage. Remember that the objectives of general massage are to get rid of excess Qi, smooth out the Qi circu-

Figure 4-4. Massage pathways on the front of the body in general massage.

Figure 4-5. Massage pathways on the back of the body in general massage.

lation, and also relax the mental and physical bodies. These goals provide the rationale for the pathways.

A. Move From Top to Bottom:

The first general rule in massage pathways is to lead the Qi downward so as to release the Qi accumulated in the head and body (Figures 4-4 and 4-5). Therefore, when you massage, your hands move from the top of the body to the bottom. If you reverse the direction, you are nourishing the Qi and leading the Qi upward. This will prevent the release of Qi and result in the body becoming more Yang, which, in turn, will cause more tension in both the mental and physical bodies.

B. Move From the Center to the Sides:

The next general rule in releasing the Qi accumulated in the body is to massage from the center of the body to the sides (Figures 4-4 and 4-5). Therefore, when you massage, your hands move from the center of the torso out to the sides. If you reverse the direction, you are nourishing the body with Qi, and preventing the release of Qi. This will result in the body becoming more Yang, and will cause more tension in both the mental and physical bodies.

C. Move in Circles:

There are many different rules for massaging in circles, and it can become very confusing. How you circle is usually more important in Tui Na, Dian Xue, and Qi massage, which are concerned with the condition of the Qi in the body. The direction of your circling determines whether you are drawing Qi in or out, and can have a great effect on whether healing takes place. The direction in which you circle is determined by the minds of the healer and the patient, and also by the channel (whether it is a Yin or Yang channel), the cavities being used, and the time of day. You can see how it is much easier to learn general massage than the healing forms of massage.

In this sub-section, we will discuss only the rules of general massage which focus on the release of mental and physical tension. If you ever become confused about which direction to circle, just take a little time to think about it, and then see the difference in how it feels to circle in either direction.

i. Leading the Qi and Blood Downward and to the Sides:

In general massage, in order to release excess Qi and improve the Qi and blood circulation, lead the Qi and blood downward to the feet and also sideways to the arms. There are a few simple rules for this.

Let us use two examples to explain these rules. First, when massaging the back of the neck, if you circle counterclockwise on the right-hand side and clockwise on the left-hand side, you are leading the Qi and blood downward (Figure 4-6). However, if you reverse the direction on both sides, then you are leading the Qi and blood upward, which may cause the head to become too Yang.

When massaging the back, if you move in a counterclockwise circle while working on the right-hand side, and in a clockwise circle while working on the left-hand side, then you are leading the Qi downward and to the sides (Figure 4-7). However, if you reverse the directions, then you are leading the Qi upward and also to the sides. If you are trying to disperse excess Qi and release tension, then you would want to bring the Qi down and to the sides. However, some-

Figure 4-6. Massage pathways on the back of the neck.

times you will want to lead Qi and blood from the back to the arms. In this case, you will circle in the other direction.

ii. Massaging the Blood and Nerve Junctions:

The blood and nerve junctions often become tense. For example, under each ear is a junction where arteries and nerves branch out and spread over the top of the head. If the top and sides of the neck are tense, the Qi and blood circulation will be affected. Massaging these junctions or knots will help the blood spread out smoothly and reduce the pressure on the junctions. Therefore, when you massage you may circle clockwise and then push upward, but you should also circle counterclockwise and then push downward (Figure 4-8). This will gently stretch the muscles around the junction and smooth out the blood and Qi circulation.

The general rule is that when you use your right hand to massage, you circle clockwise to spread the Qi and blood upward or to the right (Figure 4-9), and counterclockwise to lead the blood and Qi downward or to the right. However, if you use your left hand to massage, a counterclockwise direction will spread the Qi and blood upward and to the left, while a clockwise direction will lead the Qi and blood downward or to the left.

3. Power:

The amount of power you use is probably the most critical factor in massage. General massage works on many places, including the

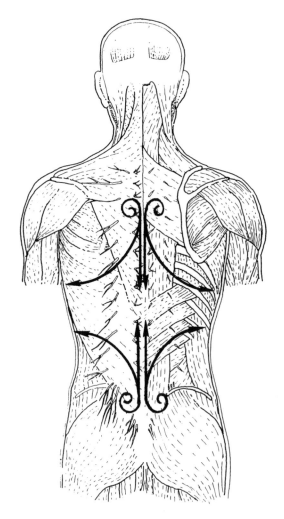

Figure 4-7. Massage pathways on the back of the body.

skin, the fascia between the skin and muscles, the fascia between muscles, the fascia between muscles and bones, the muscles themselves, the tendons around the joints, the internal organs, and the bone marrow. Massage depth ranges from the surface of the body to deep inside it. How you reach these places depends not just on the techniques you use, but also on the power you apply.

The main rule in general massage is to relax your partner. If you use too much power and cause pain, your partner will tense up, and their mind will become upset. However, if you use too little power, the massage will not be effective.

There are a few general rules which will help you reach your goals. First, the power and the pattern of the massage should be consistent. This way your partner will know what to expect, and they will be able to relax more easily. Second, start massaging lightly, and gradually increase the power. Light power gently stimulates the nerves and soothes them, so that they will not so quick to send messages to the brain. Then you can use more power without

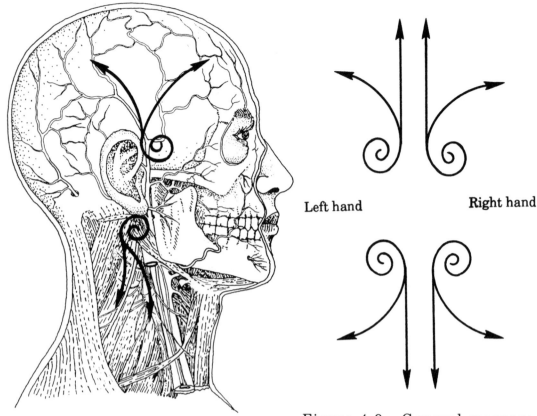

Left hand   Right hand

Figure 4-9. General massage
pathways.

Figure 4-8. Massage pathways near the ear.

disturbing your partner. Third, massage from shallow to deep. As
you stimulate the outer layers of your partner's body, the reaction of
the nerves will slow down, and their body can remain relaxed as you
increase the power and reach a deeper layer.

Fourth, finish up from deep to shallow. Once your power can
reach deep inside and remove the Qi and blood stagnation, you want
to lead this accumulated Qi, blood, and acid to the surface of the skin
and spread it out.

Finally, in order to keep the massage soft and enjoyable, your
hands must be relaxed. The trick of doing this is, when you use your
fingers to massage, generate the power and motion from your wrist
(Figure 4-10), and when you use the palm or the base of the palm to
massage, generate the power from your elbow and shoulder (Figure
4-11). If you try to generate power from the part of your body that
your are massaging with, it will be tense, and you will not be able to
apply the techniques gently. The best way to massage it to use your
entire body to generate power, and not rely on muscular power. In
addition to being the most effective way to massage, this is also very
enjoyable for you, because you can feel your whole body moving harmoniously, and you won't tire out as quickly.

Figure 4-10.

Figure 4-11.

Chapter 5
General Massage

5-1. Introduction

In this and the next chapter we will introduce the "how" of general massage. As you practice massage, many questions will occur to you, such as: 1. What are the general problems which prevent us from reaching our goals? 2. How do we solve these problems? 3. Do we get the results that the theory leads us to expect? If you keep these questions in mind as you massage, you will be able to evaluate your progress and modify your approach as necessary. In Chapter 3 we introduced many massage techniques. You may try these techniques as you practice, or even create others.

We will first introduce the mental techniques of general massage. They are used to calm down your partner, and help them relax both mentally and physically. We will then discuss the physical aspect of general massage by dividing it into five sections: the head, the back, the back of the limbs, the chest and abdomen, and the front of the limbs. In the first part of this book we discussed the general environmental requirements for massage. It is important to create a relaxed, comfortable atmosphere for you and your massage partner; I urge you to study that section carefully.

In general massage with a partner, an entire body massage usually takes about two hours. While this is very enjoyable for your partner, it requires a masseur with a lot of patience and enthusiasm. Most of the time, only part of the whole routine is done, centering on what your partner needs. The head and back are the areas which most often need treatment. The next most common areas are the legs and arms, followed by the chest and upper abdomen. The lower abdominal area is rarely treated, simply because it is near the sexual organs, and most people would feel uncomfortable unless they had a close relationship with the masseur.

When you massage your partner's whole body, if they are not shy it is best if they disrobe. This will make for the best Qi communication. Usually a towel is used to cover the areas you are not working on so that the person does not catch a cold. Many people like to wear shorts when they are being massaged. This is somewhat inconvenient when you massage the lower abdomen and the hips. When you give a general massage on only a portion of the body, it is best to expose the area you will be working on. This will help you to exchange Qi with your partner, and will give you more sensitivity in your hands. However, it is not necessary that you do this, and if your partner is reluctant to expose some part of his or her body, you needn't insist upon it.

Because general massage is not meant to treat injuries, herbal wines or ointments are not usually used. Some people use oil when they massage, such as baby oil or olive oil, on areas other than the head. While this can lubricate the skin and allow the hands to move more smoothly over it, it also seals the pores. This can interfere with the Qi communication between you and the person you are massaging. Because of this, many professional Chinese masseurs do not like to use any oil. Instead, they will often use a thin silk handkerchief to smooth the movement.

Before we introduce general massage, we would first like to discuss what the patient lies upon, be it the floor, a bed, or a specially designed wooden table. The first concern is the material beneath the patient. If you are massaging on the floor, you will need a material which provides good Qi insulation between the patient and the floor. It is best if it is made from natural materials such as cotton or wool. The thickness of the insulation is very important. If the insulation is too thin, the patient will continue to feel the Yin side of the ground and continue to lose Qi to the floor. If the material is made of synthetic material such as polyester, static charges will accumulate and make the patient feel uncomfortable. A futon is one of the most popular materials for massage, as well as for sleep and meditation.

If you use a bed for massage, it should not be too soft, which would be bad for spine massage. Padded, wooden massage tables of many different designs are available today, and are very popular (Figure 5-1).

The second concern is the neck area. When a person is lying face down on a flat surface, the head needs to be turned to the side. After a while, the neck muscles become tense and sore, and the patient is very uncomfortable. Because of this, many massage tables have an attachment which allows the patient to lie comfortably face down (Figure 5-2).

The third concern is the height of the massage table. If the table is too high, it will be difficult to massage the spine. You want to apply power easily and evenly, and it is especially important that the power of your press be even on both sides of the spinal joints. Therefore, you should be able to lower the table so that you may straddle the patient when you work on their back (Figure 5-3). However, when you massage other places such as the trunk muscles, the thighs, or the chest and abdomen, you would like the table to be

Figure 5-1. Massage table.

Figure 5-2. Head extension for a massage table.

Figure 5-3.

Figure 5-4.

about waist height so that you don't have to bend over all the time (Figure 5-4). The table needs to be the right height for you, so that you can use your whole body as you massage without expending too much effort. The best solution is a table with adjustable legs.

5-2. Massaging the Mental Body

As we explained earlier, **THE BEST RESULTS ARE OBTAINED WHEN THE PERSON BEING MASSAGED ALSO USES THEIR OWN MIND TO REGULATE THEIR BODY AND QI.** Therefore, the first step in massage is to massage the partner's

Figure 5-5.

Figure 5-6.

mind and spirit. Once you have reached their spirit, you may lead it into a deep meditative and hypnotic state. This will let their thoughts be free and their mind relaxed. Their physical body will also be relaxed, allowing you to massage and regulate their Qi and blood effectively.

When you massage your partner's mind, there are a few things that you must do. First, make your partner feel relaxed and comfortable. This involves the ambiance of your surroundings as well as to the relationship between you and your partner. Your partner needs to be able to relax totally so that they can pay attention to the condition of their body and enter a meditative state.

Next, you should draw your partner's mind away from all outside distractions and into total concentration on their body. Their attention should be totally on their Qi and your massage. There are two common ways to reach this goal. One is to ask your partner to lie face down, close their eyes, and try to relax as much as possible, and then lightly brush your hands over their body along the massage pathways, from the top of the body to the bottom, and from the center to the limbs (Figure 5-5). Repeat this several times. Then have your partner turn face upward and repeat the same process several times (Figure 5-6). Make sure that, before you actually lay your hands on them, you rub your hands together until they are warm. Few things are more startling than cold hands on your skin. Once you have brushed your partner down a few times, it will be very easy for you to bring their attention to your hands.

Some people use a different method. Instead of lightly brushing their hands over the person, they lightly slap or hit the body along the massage pathways mentioned earlier (Figure 5-7). However, according to my experience, this method is not as efficient as the previous one.

The last step of the mental massage is to massage your partner's spiritual center. The spiritual center is in the forehead, in a place called the "Shang Dan Tian" (Upper Elixir Field) by Chinese

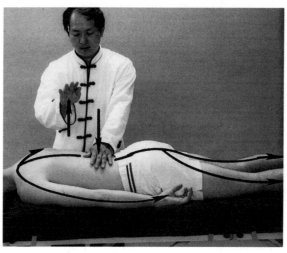

Figure 5-7.

Qigong practitioners, and the "third eye" by practitioners in the Western world. People in both Western and Asian cultures have recognized that this area can sense natural energy, and it is the center and headquarters of your spirit. With regard to physical structure, this spot is the gap between the two lobes of the brain (Figure 5-8). It is believed in Chinese Qigong that the Qi in your brain is able to reach the outside world through this center, enabling you to sense and communicate with the natural energy. Some people who train this area are able to develop their intuition and their ability to sense things that other people cannot - almost as if they could see through an extra, special eye. Therefore, the Upper Dan Tian or third eye is considered to be the gate which allows you to reach the mental center and calm down the mind.

Another common approach when massaging the Upper Dan Tian is to also stimulate the Renzhong cavity under the nose (Figure 5-8). Chinese physicians and Qigong practitioners know that stimulating the Renzhong cavity will raise the spirit of vitality and revive someone who has fainted. In massage, stimulating this cavity together with the Upper Dan Tian will help you to lead your partner's mind more easily to their center.

To massage your partner's spiritual center and Renzhong, help your partner to sit up, and let their head lean comfortably against your body. Then use your fingers or the center of your palm to massage the third eye or Upper Dan Tian slowly and gently, and at the same time press the Renzhong cavity firmly with the second or middle finger of the other hand (Figure 5-9). You may also do this when your partner is lying down (Figure 5-10).

While you are massaging their spiritual center, you should ask your partner to pay attention to your hands, relax their physical body as deeply as possible, and inhale and exhale deeply. This helps to bring them into a self-hypnotic state. People who have trained in meditation will be able to do this more easily. After mas-

Figure 5-8. The Shang Dan Tian (Upper Dan Tian) and the Renzhong cavity.

Figure 5-9.

Figure 5-10.

saging the Upper Dan Tian for a few minutes, you should be able to bring your partner into some level of meditation. Naturally, their cooperation is crucial in this.

Once you have led your partner into a meditative state, you can then start to massage their physical and Qi bodies. In the following sections, we will discuss the massage techniques for the head, back, back of the limbs, chest and abdomen, and the front of the limbs. In each section, we will first discuss the anatomical structure of the part being massaged, follow with massage theory, introduce the gates or junctions, and finally explain the massage techniques.

5-3. Massaging the Head

We mentioned earlier that the head is the most important part of the body, and should be massaged first in general massage. This discussion will also include the neck, which is the passageway to the head for Qi and blood.

Anatomical Structure of the Head and Its Circulatory Systems:

When we first look at the head, what we see is the hair or the skin. Under the surface is a layer of fat. Qi, oxygen, and nutrition are supplied to the hair and the skin by thousands of small capillaries and Qi branches. The skin also contains countless small nerves, which enable the brain to monitor the condition of the skin.

Next to the skin is the fascia. Fascia tissue can usually be found beneath the skin, between and around the muscles, between the muscles and bones, and between and around other structures such as internal organs. Under the fascia, we can see muscles, nerves, arteries, veins, lymphatics and glands. The muscles on the top of the head are usually very thin, but get thicker with different sets of muscles on the face area in order to control the movements of the eyes, nose, and mouth. Beneath the muscle is the skeleton, and again under the skeleton are many arteries, veins, and nerves which are connected to the brain.

When we look at the front of the head, under the neck muscles are large arteries, nerves, veins, lymphatics and glands, and behind them is the throat (Figure 5-11). On the side of the neck are many large sets of muscles, and underneath these muscles are big arteries, veins, and nerves (Figure 5-12). As you can see from the picture, all of the circulatory systems originate under the base of the neck, and extend to the brain and also to the top of the head.

When you look at the back of the head and neck, again you will see many arteries, veins, and nerves extending their networks from the neck to the top of the head (Figure 5-13). On the back of the neck, the spine is in the center with two large sets of muscles beside it. On each of the joints of the spine there are again arteries, veins, and nerves extending from the spinal cord to the surface of the muscles.

Remember that all of these circulatory systems are physical and therefore visible. However, in order to function, these physical systems need an invisible system to supply Qi or bioelectricity. Figures 5-14, 5-15, and 5-16 show the front, side, and back and top of the Qi circulatory system of the head.

Theory:

The head is the center of your entire being, and it governs and influences your mental body, Qi body, and physical body. When you massage the head first and relax it, your partner's mind will become calm, and their entire body will stay relaxed.

A brain cell needs 10 times as much oxygen as any other cell. When you massage the head correctly you relax the muscles and soothe the nervous system. This lets the blood vessels expand and increases the flow of blood, thereby bringing the required oxygen.

In addition, when the muscles and the nerve network in the head are relaxed, the Qi channels will be wide open and the Qi will

Figure 5-11.
Anatomical structure of
the head (front view).

Figure 5-12.
Anatomical structure of
the head (side view).

Figure 5-14. Primary Qi channels and acupuncture cavities on the head (front view).

Figure 5-13. Anatomical structure of the head (back view).

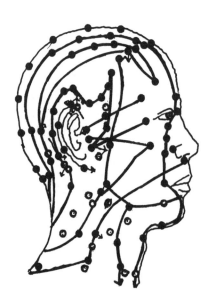

Figure 5-15. Primary Qi channels and acupuncture cavities on the head (side view).

Figure 5-16. Primary Qi channels and acupuncture cavities on the head (back view).

be able to circulate smoothly in the brain. Smooth Qi and blood circulation can prevent or even cure headaches. In addition, giving the brain cells enough Qi will slow down the natural process of degeneration. Chinese Qigong practitioners believe that the first requirement for a healthy body is to keep the brain cells healthy.

When your brain cells obtain enough oxygen and Qi, you will also be able to think more clearly. This, in turn, will increase the Qi nourishment to your spirit and raise your spirit of vitality, which is the key to longevity and health.

In massage, the head is divided into three sections: 1. the top, sides, and back of the head, 2. the face, and 3. the neck. The first section contains, as we have just seen, many nerves, blood vessels, and Qi channels hidden in the thin layer of muscle between the skin and the skull. If the nerves are tense for any reason, the muscles will tense up and hinder the smooth circulation of Qi and blood to the brain. This will result in a deficiency of Qi and blood on the top and the sides of the head, and the skin and hair will not receive the proper amount of Qi and nutrition. This deficiency is believed to be one of the main causes of gray hair and baldness.

Massaging the second section, the face, helps to keep the eyes and ears functioning well. These two senses tend to gradually fail as we get older. Massaging the face may also increase the Qi and blood circulation to the nose and mouth areas and keep them working normally.

Finally, the neck is the passageway or gate to the head for the Qi and blood. Anatomically, the neck consists of a center of bone, surrounded by many layers of muscle. Sandwiched between the layers of muscle are nerves, Qi channels, and blood vessels. The goal of massaging the neck is to relax the neck and open all of the channels and vessels.

Figure 5-17. The Baihui, Biliang, and Renzhong cavities.

In addition to the gate of the neck, there are many other small gates or pathways in the head. When you massage the head, you should focus on massaging and releasing the tension in these gates. They are the places where the Qi and blood can be blocked, causing problems such as headache (excess Qi and blood) or dizziness (deficient Qi and blood). Next, we will discuss the gates in the head.

Gates:
1. Biliang:
Biliang is not an acupuncture cavity, but it is an important gate in massage. The gate at the bridge of the nose is connected to your frontal sinuses, where your Upper Dan Tian is located (Figure 5-17). When you have a sinus problem, you get a stuffy nose. When this happens, you can lightly massage the bridge of the nose to relax the muscles around the sinuses and nose, which will often relax the nerves there. When you have difficulty breathing, your Upper Dan Tian is disturbed and your mind will not be clear.

The bridge of the nose is right over the nasal cavity, through which air enters and leaves your body. When this area is tense, the membrane inside the nose will swell and interfere with the free flow of air. This is usually what happens when you have a cold.

The most common way to massage the bridge of the nose is to use both index fingers or middle fingers to lightly press the sides of the bridge of the nose and circle around. The circle should move in toward the center on the top of the nose, and out on the bottom, and then move up to the Upper Dan Tian (Figure 5-18). This leads the Qi upward to the forehead and then allows it to be spread upward or to the sides. Usually you circle a few times on the bridge of the nose and then lead the Qi up to the Upper Dan Tian.

Figure 5-18.   Figure 5-19.

Next, again use the middle finger to circle the bridge of the nose several times in the same direction mentioned, then lead the hands downward along the sides of the nose (Figure 5-19). Finally, spread the Qi to the sides of the face.

When you do this massage, your touch must be soft. Remember: **A SOFT TOUCH HELPS RELAXATION, A HARDER PRESS WILL TENSE UP THE MUSCLES**. The motion should be smooth and continuous. This enables you to lead your partner's mind to follow your massage, and helps them to use their own Yi to lead their Qi.

2.   Renzhong (Gv-26):

The Renzhong (Philtrum) cavity under the nose is well known to Chinese physicians and Qigong practitioners for its ability to stimulate awareness and wake people up (Figure 5-17). Stimulating this cavity will raise the Qi of the head and stop a sneeze, and it can raise the spirit and immediately revive a person out of a fainting spell. Massaging the Renzhong cavity will open blockage of the Qi channels in the head.

To massage the Renzhong, simply use the thumb or the tip of the middle finger to gently press inward firmly and vibrate (Figure 5-20).

3.   Baihui (Gv-20):

Baihui (Hundred Meetings) is the cavity or Qi gate on the top of the head which allows the brain to communicate with the Qi of nature (Figure 5-17). Qi can reach the brain easily through this gate to nourish the brain.

To massage this gate, simply place the center of your right palm on the crown of the head and gently circle your hand clockwise to nourish the brain (Figure 5-21). Reversing the direction and circling counterclockwise will release Qi from the brain and relieve a headache.

Figure 5-21.

Figure 5-20.

Taiyang
(M-HN-9)

Qubin
(GB-7)

Ermen
(TB-21)

Xiaquan (S-7)

Yifeng (TB-17)

Figure 5-22. The Taiyang, Qubin, Ermen, Xiaquan, and Yifeng cavities.

4. Taiyang (M-HN-9):

The Taiyang (Sun) cavities are also known as the temples (Figure 5-22). Whenever your brain gets fatigued from too much worry or thinking, the muscles in the temple area will tense up. This can disturb the supply of Qi and blood and cause a headache. It is therefore important to open this gate by lightly massaging the temple areas to loosen up the muscles, and let the blood circulate.

The index and middle fingers are usually used to massage the temples with a circular motion. When you massage the temples, you should circle down to the neck and then to your partner's front and up to the head and finally to the back with a gentle and soft power

Figure 5-23.   Figure 5-24.

(Figure 5-23). After you have circled a few times, move the massage downward to the chin to dissipate the Qi and blood from the temples. You may repeat the process several times to release the pressure in the temple areas.

5.   Yifeng (TB-17):

The two Yifeng (Shielding Wind) cavities are very important gates which are located under the ears. A major artery runs below each ear on its way to the brain (Figure 5-22). Whenever the muscles on the sides of the neck are tight, the arteries will be constricted and the brain will not receive enough oxygen. This will cause dizziness. Constriction here may also hinder the blood returning from the head to the heart and cause headache.

Massage with your thumbs or middle finger in a circular motion, up the front and down the back (Figure 5-24). This will spread the stagnant Qi backward to the neck muscles. After circling a few times, push downward to the bottom of the neck. Repeat the process several times until you feel the areas under the ears relax.

6.   Ermen (TB-21):

Ermen (Ear's Door), which is located in front of the ear, is on the artery coming from the Yifeng cavity (Figure 5-22). In massage, the Yifeng, Ermen, and Qubin cavities are frequently treated as one, since they are all in a line on the main artery.

While the Yifeng cavity is massaged downward, Ermen and Qubin are massaged upward to the top of the head. This helps in the blood distribution from the ears to the top of the head. To massage Ermen, simply use the middle finger or the second and middle fingers to gently rub the cavity with a circular motion a few times, and then gently push upward. Pass through Qubin and rub it

Figure 5-25.   Figure 5-26.

a few times, and finish by pushing upward to lead the Qi and blood to the top of the head (Figure 5-25). When you circle, the direction should be downward to the neck, toward the back of the neck, upward, and finally forward. This will easily lead the accumulated Qi and blood upward to the top of the head.

7.   Qubin (GB-7):

As mentioned above, Qubin (Crook of the Temple) is commonly treated together with Yifeng and Ermen (Figure 5-22). The Chinese believe that when a person is getting old and gray hairs are starting to appear on the sides of the head, it is because the blood and Qi are not circulating smoothly through these three cavities. See the above paragraph for the procedure for massaging this cavity.

8.   Xiaguan (S-7):

Xiaguan (Lower Hinge) is located on the joint of the jaw (Figure 5-22). Massaging Xiaguan can remove any Qi and blood stagnation in the jaw joint, and also maintain the normal functioning of the parotid gland. To massage Xiaguan, use the index and middle fingers to rub the cavity with a circular motion. Rub up and to the rear of the head, and down and forward (Figure 5-26). Circle a few times, and then gently push downward to the chin.

9.   Tianzhu (B-10):

Tianzhu means "Heaven's Pillar," with "heaven" referring to the head. Tianzhu is located on the back of the neck (Figure 5-27).

The neck is the gate through which Qi and blood move from the body to the head, and any tension there will interfere with this circulation. You have to massage the neck and loosen up the muscles before the head can be really relaxed.

Figure 5-27. The Naohu, Tianzhu, and Jianjing cavities.

Figure 5-28.

There are two major sets of muscles in the back of the neck which support your head. When you massage the neck, most of your attention should be on these two sets of muscles. Although there are some muscles on the side of the neck, they only turn the head, and you do not need to spend too much time with them. A light, brief massage here will be sufficient to help your partner relax more fully. You can lightly touch the front of the neck and move your hand over it, but do not massage it, since there are no major muscles there.

When you massage the Tianzhu cavities, you will be able to loosen the muscles on the neck easily. Tianzhu is always massaged together with the cavity Naohu, which will be discussed next. When you massage the Tianzhu cavity, if your partner is sitting, you may use your thumbs to gently press the cavities and then circle a few times, and finally push gently downward to the back of the body. The direction of the circle should be downward at the center of the neck, then sideways, upward and then toward the center (Figure 5-28). Alternatively, you may use one of your hands to stabilize your partner's head while using the edge of the other hand to massage Tianzhu in the direction mentioned above (Figure 5-29).

You can usually achieve maximum relaxation of the neck by massaging it with your partner lying on their back. Since the neck muscles are not supporting the head, they are already relaxed. Sit or kneel above your partner's head and gently press upward on the cavities with your index and middle fingers. Move your fingers in a circular motion in the direction mentioned above and then lead the Qi sideward to the shoulders (Figure 5-30).

10. Naohu (Gv-17):

Naohu means "Brain's Household." This cavity is located in the middle of the back of the neck, between the two main muscles and just

Figure 5-30.

Figure 5-29.

under the skeleton (Figure 5-27). It is called "Brain's Household" because it is the entrance through which Qi enters the brain. Massaging this door and relaxing the muscles there is believed to improve Qi communication between the brain and the body.

To massage this cavity, simply use your right thumb (when your partner is sitting) or the right middle finger (when partner is lying down) to gently press the cavity with a circular rubbing motion (Figure 5-31). The clockwise direction is for nourishment, while counterclockwise is for releasing.

These ten gates should be done first when you massage the head. If the muscles around these gates remain tense, the Qi and blood circulation will be affected. When you massage these gates, do not cause any pain, since this will only make the muscles more tense. Simply massage them lightly in the appropriate direction before you start massaging the pathways. Remember to rub your hands together until they are warm before you touch your partner.

Massaging the Head

Next, we will introduce some of the common massage techniques and pathways on the head which are used in general massage. There are two common positions which can be used to massage the head: sitting, and lying face upward.

1. With your Partner Sitting:

Your partner can sit cross-legged on the floor, with you kneeling behind; or in a chair, with you standing behind them. Your partner should be as comfortable as possible. If you let your partner lean their head against you, they will be able to relax their head and spine (Figure 5-32).

Figure 5-31.

Figure 5-32.

Step #1:

Gently massage the bridge of the nose with your middle fingers in a circular motion about five times. Circle according to the rules discussed earlier. Then stroke the fingers upward to the center of the forehead. Finally, gently stroke your hands to the top of your partner's head, down the back of the neck, and out to the sides (Figure 5-33). Do this five to ten times. This path smoothes out the superficial circulation of the Qi and blood in the head. In order to lead the Qi out of the neck and head, after you complete each movement, grab the Jianjing cavity (i.e., Shoulder Well) with the thumb and all of the fingers and massage the muscles there (Figure 5-34). This will lead the Qi further out to the shoulders from the neck area. You may also massage the Gaohuang cavity on the back and lead the Qi from the neck to the back (Figure 5-35). The Jianjing and Gaohuang cavities are important gates in back massage.

After you have completed this massage pathway, again circle the bridge of the nose with your middle fingers in the same direction and then gently press and brush downward along the sides of the nose. Repeat several times. Finally, use your fingers to spread from the nose area to the cheeks (Figure 5-36).

This massage will release tension in the sinus area, improve the Qi and blood circulation there, and spread the accumulated Qi and blood both upward and downward.

Step #2:

Again circle your middle fingers on the bridge of your partner's nose about five times, and then move them up to the forehead. Brush with your middle and index fingers to the sides of the forehead, circle a few times on the temples (Taiyang), brush down to the

Figure 5-33.

Figure 5-34.

Figure 5-35.

Figure 5-36.

jaws and circle a few times, and finally brush down the front of the neck to the chest (Figure 5-37). Repeat the procedure five to ten times. This pathway can relax the temple and jaw areas and improve Qi and blood circulation in the face.

Step #3:

Again start at the bridge of the nose. Circle your middle fingers five times, and then use your index and middle fingers to gently circle the eyes about five times. Finally, rub to the sides of the eyes and downward to the jaw (Figure 5-38). Repeat the procedure about

Figure 5-37.

Figure 5-38.

Figure 5-39.

Figure 5-40.

five to ten times. Then rub your hands together until they are warm, and gently place the base of your palms on your partner's eyes to nourish them with the Qi from your palms (Figure 5-39). Then stroke sideward with the base of the palms to the temples and downward to the cheeks (Figure 5-40). This is called "ironing the eyes" (Tang Yan). This path improves the Qi and blood circulation around the eyes and slows the deterioration of the eyes.

Step #4:

Gently press your index fingers in front of your partner's ears on the Ermen cavity, and rub lightly up and around the ears until your

Figure 5-41.

Figure 5-42.

Figure 5-43.

Figure 5-44.

fingers reach the bottom of the ears, then stroke downward to the sides of the neck (Figure 5-41). Do this about five times. Next, press your hands on their ears, then circle the ears five times in one direction and then five times in the other direction (Figure 5-42). Next, press the ears and immediately release several times to pop the ears (Figure 5-43). Finally, massage the entire ear with your fingers (Figure 5-44). According to Chinese medicine, different portions of the ears correspond to different internal organs. Massaging the ears can stimulate and improve the functioning of the internal organs. This massaging path can also keep the ears functioning properly.

Figure 5-45.   Figure 5-46.

Step #5:

Next, massage the muscles on the back of the neck, especially in the areas of the gates. When you massage the back of the neck, let your partner's head lean slightly backward to relax the muscles. Starting at the base of the skull, press and push with your thumbs down along the neck muscles on both sides of the spine (Figure 5-45). Alternatively, you may change your massage position and use one of your hands to support your partner's head by pressing gently forward on their forehead and using the edge of the other hand to gently rub downward on the back of the neck (Figure 5-46). Repeat ten times.

Then use the thumb and fingers of one hand to grab and rub the back of the neck ten times, paying particular attention to the Tianzhu and Naohu cavities. This loosens up the neck, and allows the Qi and blood to pass through the neck more smoothly. However, you also need to lead any excess Qi down out of the head so that it doesn't stagnate there. Therefore, you should again grab and massage the shoulder muscles (Jianjing cavity) on both sides with your fingers (Figure 5-47). Naturally, you may again lead the Qi to the back by massaging the Gaohuang cavity on the back (Figure 5-48).

Step #6:

This is the final pathway for massaging the head. After you have loosened up all of the gates and muscles on the head and neck, you now want to lead the Qi accumulated under the skin and in the muscles to the surface of the skin so that you can lead it downward to the neck and spread it out to the back of the body.

The first way to do this is to loosen up the fasciae between the skin and the skeleton. Simply place one or both palms on your partner's head. Gently press downward and move the skin in a circular motion (Figure 5-49). After circling a few times, stroke down-

Figure 5-47.

Figure 5-48.

Figure 5-49.

Figure 5-50.

ward. Circle toward the center and downward to the back of the neck (Figure 5-50). You may also circle in the other direction to lead the Qi downward from the forehead to the face, however, experience shows that it is better to lead the Qi backward instead of forward.

Next, gently tap your fingertips over the entire head (Figure 5-51). This will lead the Qi to the surface of the skin. When you tap, you should always start at the center and move to the sides and back. After you finish tapping, again use your palms to brush the head from the top to the back of the neck and finally down to the shoulder and the back of the body.

Figure 5-52.

Figure 5-51.

2.   With your Partner Lying Down:

When you massage the neck, you may also have your partner lie on their back. This position has several advantages compared to the sitting position. First, the neck muscles can be very relaxed simply because they don't have to support the head. This allows you to penetrate more deeply into the neck. Second, lying down is more relaxed and more comfortable for the person being massaged, and therefore the massage can be more enjoyable.

When you massage someone who is lying down, you cannot always use the same techniques that you use when they are sitting, and sometimes you will use different parts of the hand to massage an area. However, whichever position you and your partner use, the goals and the theory of the massage remain the same.

When you massage, you should be sitting or kneeling comfortably above their head. If they are undressed, you should cover their body with a towel to keep them warm.

Step #1:

Use your thumbs to gently massage the bridge of your partner's nose about five times with a circular motion (Figure 5-52). The direction of the circle should follow the rules discussed in the section on pathways in Chapter 4. Then stroke the thumbs upward to the center of the forehead. Finally, gently stroke your hands to the sides of your partner's head, circle a few times on the temples (Figure 5-53) and down the sides of their neck, and then out to the chest (Figure 5-54). Do this five to ten times.

After you have completed this pathway, again use your thumbs or middle finger to circle the bridge of the nose in the same direction, and then gently press and brush downward along the sides of the

Figure 5-53.

Figure 5-54.

Figure 5-55.

Figure 5-56.

nose. Finally, use your hands to spread from the nose area to the cheeks (Figure 5-55). Repeat several times.

This massage will release tension in the sinus area, improve Qi and blood circulation there, and disperse the accumulated Qi and blood both upward and downward.

Step #2:

Again start at the bridge of the nose. Circle your thumbs five times, and then use your thumbs to gently circle the eyes about five times (Figure 5-56). Finally, rub to the sides of the eyes and downward to the jaw (Figure 5-57). Repeat the procedure five to ten times. Then rub your hands together until they are warm, and gently place the base of your thumbs on their eyes to nourish them with the Qi from your palms (Figure 5-58). Then stroke sideward with the base of the thumbs to the temples and downward to the cheeks (Figure 5-59).

Figure 5-57.

Figure 5-58.

Figure 5-59.

Figure 5-60.

Step #3:

Gently press your index fingers in front of your partner's ears on the Ermen cavity, and rub lightly up and around the ears until your fingers reach the bottoms of the ears, then stroke downward to the sides of the neck (Figure 5-60). Do this about five times. Next, press your hands on their ears, then circle the ears five times in one direction and then five times in the other direction (Figure 5-61). Then press on the ears and immediately release the pressure to pop the ears a few times (Figure 5-62). Finally, massage the entire ear with your fingers (Figure 5-63).

Step #4:

Use your fingers to lift and rub the muscles on the back of the neck, especially on the gates (Figure 5-64). After you have loosened up the neck muscles, you also need to lead any excess Qi down out of the head so that it doesn't stagnate there. Therefore, grab and

Figure 5-61.

Figure 5-62.

Figure 5-63.

Figure 5-64.

massage the shoulder muscles again (Jianjing cavity) on both sides (Figure 5-65). Finally, use your hands to stroke and brush from the neck to the shoulders (Figure 5-66).

Step #5:

After you have loosened up all of the gates and muscles on the head and neck, you then want to loosen up the fasciae between the skin and the skeleton. Place one or both palms on your partner's head, press downward gently, and move the skin in a circular motion (Figure 5-67). After circling a few times, stroke to the sides and then downward. Finally, brush with your hands from the back of the neck to the shoulders and the chest.

5-4. Massaging the Back

The back, in this discussion, runs from the base of the neck down to the coccyx, and to the sides of the body from the armpit to

Figure 5-65.

Figure 5-66.

Figure 5-67.

the waist. Below the sides of the waist and the sacrum is considered to be part of the legs, and will be discussed in the next section.

Anatomical Structure of the Back and Its Circulatory Systems:

Underneath the skin of the back are many sets of muscles and many nerves branching out from the center to the sides (Figure 5-68).

Beneath the muscles are the spine and ribs (Figure 5-69), with many nerves (PNS) branching out from the spine. The nerves from the neck vertebrae spread out to the arms, while the nerves from the lower portion of the spinal cord extend to the legs. The nerves from the middle section of the spine (the thoracic vertebrae) branch out and reach to the various internal organs.

Behind the ribs on the upper section of the back are the lungs. Behind the lowest ribs are the kidneys. Many nerves branch out to the hip area, and a big nerve passes through the pelvis to the back of the thighs.

Figure 5-68. Superficial anatomical structure of the posterior aspect of the trunk.

Figure 5-69. Deep anatomical structure of the posterior aspect of the trunk.

Theory:

The spine is the center of the nervous system, with nerves extending out to the brain, the limbs, and the internal organs (Figure 5-69). It is through this network that the brain controls the body.

From the point of view of Qi, the Governing Vessel runs along the back of the spine, and the Thrusting Vessel is inside the spinal cord (Figure 5-70). According to Chinese medicine and Qigong, the Governing Vessel is the Qi reservoir which supplies and regulates the Qi circulation in the six primary Yang channels, while the Thrusting Vessel is the reservoir which nourishes the Qi in the spinal cord and brain. The nervous system is constructed of physical cells which need to be nourished with Qi (bioelectricity) to function and stay alive. This tells us that Qi is ultimately responsible for the functioning of the nerves.

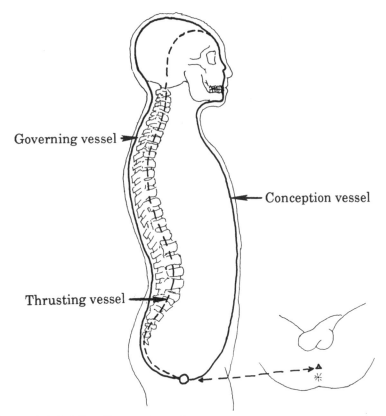

Figure 5-70. The Governing, Conception, and Thrusting vessels.

The spine is the center of our Qi distribution system, and also of our ability to sense our surroundings. If the muscles around the spine remain tense, the Qi circulation and the functioning of the nerves can be affected in the whole body. Therefore, right after massaging the head, you should massage the spine and loosen up the muscles around it.

While your entire body is supported by the spine, the ability to move your body depends upon the four sets of large trunk muscles, two in the front of your body, and two in the back. Whenever these muscles are tense, your trunk will be tense, and the Qi circulation along and in the spine will be affected. Therefore, when you massage the back, you must pay particular attention to loosening up the two trunk muscles on the sides of the spine. This will also relax the kidneys beneath the muscles, and improve the Qi circulation in them.

When you massage the back, therefore, you must first focus on the spinal area, and lead the Qi downward to the sacrum and spread it out to the hips and legs. You must also spread the Qi in the center of the back out to the sides (Figure 5-71). Next, you will focus on the trunk muscles in the back. The rule is to first lead the Qi from deep inside the body to the surface, and then spread it out from the top to the bottom and from the center to the sides.

Before we discuss the gates, let us first review the Qi channels in the back. As mentioned earlier, the Governing Vessel is in the center

Figure 5-71. Massage pathways on the back of the body in general massage.

of the back along the outside of the spine, and the Thrusting Vessel is inside the spine. The Qi circulating in the Governing Vessel is used to nourish the Yang channels and the development of the physical body, while the Thrusting Vessel nourishes the marrow and the brain. In addition to the cavities on these two vessels, there are thirty-eight miscellaneous cavities (M-BW-1 to M-BW-38) on the sides of the vertebrae where the nerves branch out from the spinal cord (Figure 5-72). Stimulating these cavities properly can relax all the nerve junctions and also affect the Qi circulation in the Governing Vessel.

On each side of these cavities are two branches of the Yang Urine Bladder channel. This channel runs straight down from the top of the head to the bottom of the feet, splitting into two parallel branches in the back (Figure 5-72). On the inner branch are cavities which are closely related to the health of the internal organs. These cavities are: Feishu (B-13)(Lung Admittance), Xinshu (B-15)(Heart Admittance), Ganshu (B-18)(Liver Admittance), Danshu (B-19)(Gall Bladder

Figure 5-72. Primary Qi channels and acupuncture cavities on the back of the body.

Admittance), Pishu (B-20)(Spleen Admittance), Weishu (B-21)(Stomach Admittance), Sanjiaoshu (B-22)(Triple Burner Admittance), Shenshu (B-23)(Kidney Admittance), and Dachangshu (B-25)(Large Intestine Admittance). Shu in Chinese means "allowance" or "admittance." Sometimes they are translated as "doors."

These cavities are related to many of the internal organs, and are the Qi entrances from the back. Actually, if you take a detailed look,

Figure 5-73. The Jianjing, Tianzong, Gaohuang, Lingtai, Mingmen, Shenshu, and Changquang cavities.

you can also see that almost all of the cavities on these channels are entrances which allow the Qi to communicate with the front of the body. All of these cavities are located on the inner branch of the Urinary Bladder channel. In order to open all of these gates or doors, the spine and the trunk muscles must first be relaxed. Next, we will discuss a number of additional gates which are also important.

Gates on the Back
1. Jianjing (GB-21):
Jianjing means "Shoulder Well" and is the passageway between the neck and the arms. Stimulating the Jianjing cavity correctly will not only open up the Qi channels from the head to the arms, but also stimulate the skin and open all the pores. Stimulating this cavity causes a very pleasant, exciting feeling in the patient, and gives them goose bumps all over the body. Jianjing is frequently used in acupuncture and Qigong to lead the Qi which has accumulated in the head to the arms, thereby relieving headaches and releasing pressure in the head.

You can see that the massage of the head does not end with the neck. Once you have loosened up the neck muscles and the Qi and blood start to circulate smoothly, you need to lead away the Qi which was accumulated there and has come up to the surface. Therefore, you should continue on to the Jianjing cavity area (Figure 5-73),

Figure 5-74.   Figure 5-75.

which will lead Qi from the neck to the shoulders and spread it out so that it can get back into circulation.

To open this gate, simply grasp the shoulder muscles with your thumb and fingers, and rub the muscles forward and backward, vibrating them gently (Figure 5-74). Do not use too much power when you do this, as it will be painful and cause the muscles to tense. This will seal the gates, rather than open them. After rubbing a few times, the shoulder muscles should be loose and more relaxed. Then press the cavity with your index and middle fingers, and make a circular motion to stimulate the cavity more deeply (Figure 5-75). Finally, slide your hands or the edge of your hands along the shoulder muscles and down to the shoulder joints (Figure 5-76).

2. Tianzong (SI-11):

The Tianzong (Heaven's Ancestor) cavity is located in the center of the shoulder blade and belongs to the small intestine channel (Figure 5-73). Tianzong is the Qi passageway between the arm and the back. In the martial arts, this cavity may be struck to paralyze the entire arm. A gentle massage, however, can open this passage and allow smooth Qi communication between the arm and the back.

To massage this cavity, use your index and middle fingers to press gently with a circular motion. If you use your right hand on the cavity located on the right, circling clockwise will lead Qi to the arms, while circling counterclockwise will lead Qi downward (Figure 5-77). You may also use the base of the palm to massage this gate.

3.   Gaohuang (B-38):

The Gaohuang (Vital's Hollow) cavity is located right beside the shoulder blade near the spine (Figure 5-73). In the martial arts, this

Figure 5-76.   Figure 5-77.

cavity is struck to contract the lungs and "seal the breath." It is believed that when this cavity is seriously injured, the Qi circulation in the heart and certain other internal organs can be affected. In China, when a person is very sick and near death, it is said "Bin Ru Gaohuang," which means that "the sickness has reached the Gaohuang." The situation is then hopeless, because when the Qi is stagnant there, death is imminent.

To massage the Gaohuang cavity, push the shoulder back slightly with one hand to loosen up the area, and then use the edge of the other hand to circle the cavity and push downward (Figure 5-78).

4.   Lingtai (Gv-10):

The Lingtai cavity, or the "Spirit's Platform," is so called because it is opposite the heart (Figure 5-73). Stimulating this cavity correctly will relax the heart. However, very strong stimulation may cause a heart attack. Massaging this cavity can balance the Qi in the front and the back of the body.

When you massage Lingtai, you should not put pressure on the bones directly and cause pain. The best way to massage this cavity is to press gently with the base of the palm or side of your fist and circle. When you circle clockwise, you are nourishing the heart. However, there is usually too much Qi in the heart, so you would normally circle in a counterclockwise direction, and then lead the Qi downward to the lower back (Figure 5-79).

5.   Mingmen (Gv-4):

Mingmen means "Life's Door." It is called this because it is the gate through which you can reach the residence of the Qi: the Lower Dan Tian. In Qigong theory, the Lower Dan Tian in your lower

Figure 5-78.

Figure 5-79.

abdomen is called "Jia Dan Tian," which means the "false Dan Tian," while the space between the false Dan Tian and the Mingmen is called "Zhen Dan Tian," or the "real Dan Tian" (Figure 5-80). While the false Dan Tian is the furnace which generates Qi, the real Dan Tian is the residence which stores the Qi which has been generated. According to Chinese medicine, Qi is the origin of life. The Mingmen is therefore the door to reach this Qi storage place.

On the sides of the Mingmen are the two Shenshu (Kidney Admittance) cavities (Figure 5-73). Massaging these two doors can improve the Qi communication between the kidneys and the surrounding environment. When you massage Mingmen, you should also massage the Shenshu cavities.

When you massage Mingmen and Shenshu to open them, you may use the base of the palm or the side of the fist to circle them. Theoretically, you would like to nourish and increase the Qi in the Qi residence, and also nourish the Qi in your kidneys, since it is usually deficient there. Therefore, when you massage these gates, your right hand should circle clockwise while the left hand should circle counterclockwise (Figure 5-81).

6. Sacrum:

In Chinese Qigong, the sacrum is the junction where the Qi enters the spinal cord and reaches up to the brain. The sacrum is called "Xian Gu," which means "immortal bone." This is because, in the advanced practices which lead the practitioner to Buddhahood or enlightenment and then immortality, the Qi must be led upward through the Thrusting Vessel in the spinal cord to reach the brain and nourish the spirit. To do this, you need to learn how to lead the Qi into the spinal cord through the sacrum.

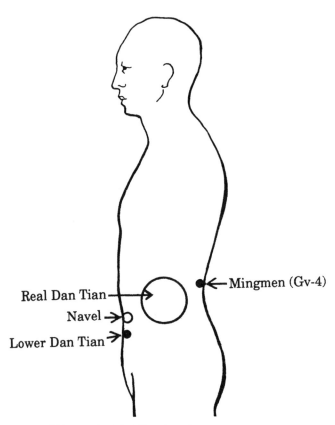

Figure 5-80. The Real Dan Tian.

Massaging the sacrum, in addition to sending a pleasant sensation to the brain, also sends Qi from the back to the bottom of the feet. This is because the sacrum connects the Qi from the legs with the Qi which goes all the way to the brain.

To massage the sacrum, use the base of your palm or the side of the fist to rub the area with a circular motion. Since this is the junction of the upward Qi and downward Qi, you should circle in both directions the same number of times (Figure 5-82).

7. Changqiang (Gv-1):

Changqiang (Long Strength) is also called "Weilu," which means "tailbone." The Changqiang cavity is the first cavity on the Yang Governing Vessel where the Qi circulation leaves the Yin Conception Vessel (Figure 5-73). It is believed in Chinese Qigong that, as you get older, this cavity seals up more and more, which interferes with normal Qi circulation in the Governing and Conception Vessels. When this happens, the Qi circulating in the twelve primary Qi channels will be affected and the Qi level in the twelve internal organs will not be regulated smoothly. It is believed that this is the cause of aging.

In the Chinese martial arts, Changqiang is one of the death cavities, and when it is struck it has a severe or even fatal effect.

When you massage the Changqiang cavity, first use the base of your palm to push inward and upward a few times (Figure 5-83).

Figure 5-81.

Figure 5-82.

Figure 5-83.

Figure 5-84.

Next, use the base of the palm or the second and middle fingers to rub the cavity gently. If you use your right hand, massage clockwise and then push upward (Figure 5-84). This will follow the natural Qi circulation which is upward to the back from the Changqiang cavity. This can also lead the Qi to the sacrum and enter the spinal cord and bone marrow in the spine.

Before you massage the entire back, you may wish to first massage each of the above gates. You may also simply use the following techniques to massage the whole back, and pay extra attention to these gates.

Massaging the Back:

After you have completed the head and neck massage, you should let your partner lie face down. Ideally, you should have a

Figure 5-85.   Figure 5-86.

massage table with a special extension for the head. If you do not, or if your partner is lying on the floor, you may place a soft pillow under their chest to keep the neck muscles relaxed, and to facilitate breathing (Figure 5-85).

Step #1:

The first thing to do when you massage the back is to lead Qi from the neck to the arms and back. If you fail to do this, even though you have loosened up the head and neck the Qi will still be in the head, and it will eventually return to the problem sites. It is therefore important to remember to lead the Qi away from the head and neck.

The first step is to grab and gently squeeze the Jianjing cavities on the muscles between the neck and the shoulders (Figure 5-86). While you are grabbing, use your thumb to press the Jianjing cavity and rub around. Finally, use your second or middle finger to press the Jianliao (TB-14) cavity located on the top of the shoulder joint (Figure 5-87). This will lead the Qi to the top of the arms and spread it out there.

Next, lift your partner's shoulder up with one hand, and rub and massage the Tianzong (SI-11) with the second and middle fingers (Figure 5-88). Continue to rub the Gaohuang (B-38) cavities with the edge of the other hand (Figure 5-89). This will lead Qi from the neck downward to the back.

Finally, use the base of your palms (Figure 5-90) to press the two back trunk muscles, moving down from the head to the lower back with a circular massaging motion. Massage both sides and repeat the same process about five times. This will loosen up the trunk muscles and release tension in the spine. Do not massage upward, because it would lead Qi back to the neck and cause problems.

Step #2:

Once you have finished the circular pressing massage of the back trunk muscles, place one hand on top of the other and press down on each joint in the spine. Do not press on the neck. Be sure that you press on the joints, and not on the vertebrae. The purpose

Figure 5-87.

Figure 5-88.

Figure 5-89.

Figure 5-90.

is to bend and loosen the joints a little (Figure 5-91). Press in coordination with your partner's breathing. Place your hands in position and ask your partner to inhale deeply and then exhale. When your partner is exhaling, press down. How hard you press depends on your partner. Start with light power and observe your partner's reaction. If they hold their breath and tense up, then you are pressing too hard. Make sure that your posture is comfortable and your power is even and firm. You may repeat the entire procedure once.

Next, starting from the neck and moving down the length of the spine, press your thumbs into the gaps between the joints to stimulate the miscellaneous cavities just beside the center of the spine (Figure 5-92). When you reach the sacrum, massage it with the base of your palm (Figure 5-93).

Figure 5-91.

Figure 5-92.

Figure 5-93.

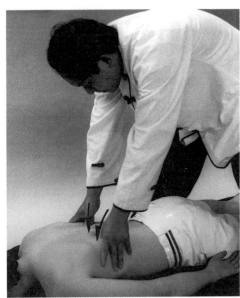

Figure 5-94.

After you have finished pressing on the sides of the spine, repeat the procedure, only now press about two inches away from the spine on the cavities on the inner branch of Urine Bladder channel (Figure 5-94). After pressing, again use the forearm, the palm, or the edge of the palm to rub the trunk muscles in small circles, pushing to the sides and also downward (Figure 5-95). This procedure leads stagnant Qi sideways and downward away from the spine. Repeat the process several times.

Step #3:

Once you have loosened up the spine and the trunk muscles,

Figure 5-95. Figure 5-96.

you should now lead the Qi to the arms, the sides of the body, and downward to the legs.

To lead the Qi to the arms, first loosen up the area of the shoulder blades. To do this, place your partner's arm behind them, then lift up the shoulder with both hands and gently move it in a circle. Move the right shoulder clockwise (Figure 5-96) and the left shoulder counterclockwise to loosen the entire shoulder area.

Next, press with your second and middle fingers on the Tianzong cavity in the center of the shoulder blade and gently rub around. To lead Qi to the arms, circle clockwise with your right hand on the right shoulder blade (Figure 5-97), and counterclockwise with your left hand on the left shoulder blade.

After you have massaged the Tianzong cavity, use your hand to brush the skin from the spine over the Tianzong cavity and out to the arms. This will lead stagnant Qi from the back to the arms.

Step #4:

You now want to spread the accumulated Qi to the sides of the back. To do this, first you may want to use the sides of your palms to hit the entire back gently from the top to the bottom and from the center to the sides (Figure 5-98). Alternatively, you may want to grab the skin on the back and shake it a little (Figure 5-99). This will bring up any Qi still hidden under the skin.

Next, brush with your hands from the top to the bottom and from the center to the sides (Figure 5-100). After brushing several times, grab the muscles under the armpits with both hands and rub and shake them (Figure 5-101). Next, use your hands to brush from the armpit areas downward to the sides of the waist.

Finally, follow the gaps in the ribs with your fingers, pushing from the center of the back to the sides (Figure 5-102). Repeat several times.

Figure 5-97.

Figure 5-98.

Figure 5-99.

Figure 5-100.

Step #5:

Finally, you want to spread the Qi downward to the legs. To do this, you must first loosen the waist area. Start with the kidneys. Good Qi circulation in the kidneys is very important. When it is abnormal, the surrounding area will also be affected.

To massage the kidneys, use a circular motion. The right hand should move clockwise on the right kidney, while the left hand should move counterclockwise on the left kidney (Figure 5-103). These circular motions will nourish the kidneys, and they can also spread the accumulated Qi to the sides of the body. When you massage the kidneys, you may also press gently down on them with

Figure 5-102.

Figure 5-101.

Figure 5-103.

Figure 5-104.

your palms, and then release the pressure (Figure 5-104). Do this about ten times and you will feel the tension in the kidneys release and the Qi circulation improve. Finally, use both palms to push from the kidneys to the sides of the body and also downward to the hips.

In order to loosen the waist area more, you may simply hold the sides of the waist with both hands and gently raise and lower it a few times (Figure 5-105).

Next, press and release with your palms on the joint between the sacrum and the first vertebra about ten times (Figure 5-106), and then push to the sides and to the hips to lead the Qi there

Figure 5-105.   Figure 5-106.

(Figure 5-107). In the next section, we will introduce the gates in the hip area which lead Qi to the legs.

5-5. Massaging the Back of the Limbs

There are twelve Qi channels in the limbs, six in the arms and the other six in the legs. The other ends of these channels are connected to the twelve internal organs. There are three Yang channels and three Yin channels in the arms, and also in the legs. Generally, the Yang channels are on the external sides of the limbs, while the Yin channels run along the internal sides. The Qi in the Yang channels is relatively stronger than the Qi in the Yin channels. Consequently, the parts of the physical body which are nourished by the Yang channels are more developed, and more able to resist outside force. The internal parts of the limbs are relatively weaker, but, because they are under less strain, the Qi flow can be smoother, and Qi disturbances on the Yin parts of the body can be sensed more easily by the brain.

For example, when you pinch or strike the external sides of the limbs you will feel less pain than you would on the internal sides. You are also more ticklish on the internal sides. Because of this, the Chinese martial arts emphasize using the external sides of the limbs for blocking, while they aim their attacks at the opponent's internal sides. This Yin and Yang theory can also apply to the torso. The front side is Yin and is more vital than the back side which is Yang.

It is important to remember this when you massage, and to use less power on the internal sides of the limbs, lest you cause bruises.

You also need to be aware of the importance of massaging the limbs. The torso contains the internal organs, which absorb the essence of food and air and convert it through a biochemical reaction into Qi. This Qi is then supplied to the entire body. However, when

Laogong
(P-8)

Figure 5-107.

Figure 5-108. The Laogong cavity.

there is an excess of Qi, or when the Qi loses its balance and affects the mutual cooperation among the organs, then the excess Qi is released through the limbs until balance is restored.

For example, your heart can be energized when you are excited. When this happens, the Qi in the heart is Yang (excessive), and the normal functioning of the heart may be impaired. The excess Qi is therefore led through the pericardium channel to the centers of your palms and released into the air. As this happens, you will feel warm and your palms will perspire. The pericardium is the membrane which encloses the heart, and is considered an organ in Chinese medicine. On the pericardium channel in the center of each palm is a cavity called Laogong (which means "labor palace"). These cavities are the main gates for regulating the condition of the heart (Figure 5-108).

There are many important cavities on the legs. For example, the Yongquan (Gushing Spring) cavities on the soles of the feet regulate the Qi in another important internal organ, the kidneys (Figure 5-109). In addition to the cavity gates, there are also thousands of pores, which are also considered gates.

In addition to acting as gates for releasing excess Qi from the organs, the limbs also play a role in Qi nourishment. Whenever you move or exercise, the food essence accumulated in your body as fat is converted into Qi and flows through the Qi channels to the internal organs. This is how Wai Dan Qigong (External Elixir Qigong) works.

In this section, we will discuss massaging the back of the limbs. Actually, we will discuss not just the back of the thighs and upper arms, but also both sides of the calves, feet, forearms, and hands. The reason for this is simply that, since the elbows and knees bend so easily, it is easy to massage the calves and forearms even when

Yongquan
(K-1)

Figure 5-109. The Yongquan cavity.

your partner is lying face down. We will start this discussion with the legs, and then cover the arms.

The front of the thighs and upper arms will be discussed after the front of the body has been dealt with. Once the chest and abdomen are massaged, the front of the body is relaxed and the Qi is flowing smoothly. The limbs should then be massaged to lead the Qi to the feet and hands.

1. Massaging the Back of the Thighs, Calves, and Feet: Anatomical Structure of the Leg and Its Circulatory Systems:

Beneath the skin on the back of the leg are the muscles, some nerves which extend from the hip to the foot, and also some veins on the back and inner side of the calf. Under a layer of muscle is the main nerve coming down from the hip, and also several smaller branches extending upward to the hip area (Figure 5-110).

In addition, the main artery runs from in front of the hip joint and extends downward to the back of the thigh, where it runs parallel to the main nerve. There are also several smaller arteries branching out from the lower hip to the center of the hip. You can see in the last two illustrations how it is possible for you to reach the main nerve and blood vessel on the back of the knee.

Beneath the last layer of muscle are the main nerves and muscles in the legs (Figure 5-110). The area around the sacrum is very important in massage because it is the main gate for Qi channels, nerves, and blood vessels into the legs.

Just beneath the skin in the front of the leg, in addition to the muscles are many nerves and some veins extending downward from the hip joint. There are also some major nerves, veins and arteries near the joint. Beneath the muscles are the main nerve and artery systems running downward to the toes (Figure 5-111).

Finally, Figures 5-112 and 5-113 show the anatomical structure of the feet from the bottom and the top. You can see that most of the nerve and blood circulatory systems are hidden in the gaps between the bones.

Figure 5-110. Anatomical structure of the posterior aspect of the leg (back view).

Theory:

The nerves connected to the legs originate in the lower portion of the spine, which, in turn, is connected to the brain. To maintain and improve the functioning of this network of nerves which connects the brain and the legs, you start by loosening up the lower part of the spine. Once you have relieved tension in the lower part of the body, the Qi will be able to circulate smoothly between the brain and the legs. Always remember, **QI IS THE ROOT AND LIFE OF THE PHYSICAL BODY.** Uneven Qi circulation will interfere with the functioning of the physical nervous system.

The hips are the gate for Qi and blood communication between the lower spine and the legs. Therefore, massaging the hips is the most important part of massaging the legs. The key to successful leg

Figure 5-111. The anatomical structure of the posterior aspect of the leg (front view).

massage is relaxing the big muscles in the hips and opening and stimulating the Qi gates in the hips.

After massaging the hips and opening the gates there, you then move down to the thighs. The thigh muscles are big and thick, and you need very strong fingers to reach the muscles deep inside. Positioning your partner's legs correctly will make it easier. For example, when you massage the thigh and the calf, lift the foot up about twelve inches; with the leg bent, the muscles and tendons will be more relaxed, and it will be easier for you to penetrate.

You may find that it is difficult for you to generate enough power when using finger techniques. If this is the case, then using your feet may prove more effective. In the first part of this book we discussed how many parts of the body could be used for giving a massage. Feel free to experiment with them, and discover which ones work best for you in various circumstances. As long as your

Figure 5-112. Anatomical structure of the posterior aspect of the foot (bottom view).

Figure 5-113. Anatomical structure of the posterior aspect of the foot (top view).

partner stays relaxed and you can achieve your massage goals, they are good techniques. Do not feel that you must restrict yourself to the techniques we mention in this chapter.

After massaging the thighs, you then move on to the calves. First massage the tendons and open the Qi gates around the knees, which are the gates between the thighs and the calves. When you massage the calf muscles, the position of the foot should be the same as when you massaged the thigh. It should be easier to massage the calf, since the muscles there are not as thick as in the thigh, and the gate cavities are shallower.

Next massage the ankles, which are the junctions between the calves and the feet, and finally massage the feet. The bottoms of the feet are more important than the tops because that is where the Yongquan cavity is located. Massaging the feet is very effective in calming people down, and can even put them to sleep.

Next, we will describe the gates on the legs, and follow this with a discussion of massage techniques. But first, please familiarize yourself with the Qi circulatory system in the legs, as shown in Figures 5-114 to 5-116.

Gates:

1. Zhongkong (M-BW-26), Zhibian (B-49), and Baihuanshu (B-30):

Zhongkong (Middle Space), Zhibian (Order's Edge), and Baihuanshu (White Circle's Hollow) are the gates which open up the Qi circulation from the lower back to the back of the thigh (Figure 5-117). Stimulating these three gates properly can generate a strong sensation which moves from the lower back to the feet. Frequently, stimulating any of these cavities will also cause the cavity on the back of the knee (Weizhong) or the Yongquan cavity on the bottom of the foot to also be stimulated. This multiple stimulation leads the Qi straight down to the knee or to the bottom of the feet.

When you massage these cavities, you may simply use your thumb, the second and middle fingers, or even the base of the palm to press firmly on the cavity and then rub around (Figure 5-118). The direction of the circle is not as critical here as elsewhere, since you are either spreading the Qi to the side or leading it downward. When you massage these cavities, start with the top one and move downward to the bottom ones. It is important not to use too much power when you massage these cavities, since any pain will cause the hip muscles to tense and hinder the massage.

In order to build up the connection, the gates on the back of the legs will often be stimulated right after the ones on the hips. Additional gates on the back of the leg are Yinmen, Weizhong, and Chengshan, which will be discussed later.

2. Jiankua (N-LE-55) and Huantiao (GB-30):

Jiankua (Strengthen Thigh) and Huantiao (Encircling Leap) are two important cavities located on the external sides of the thighs, and which are the gates which connect the waist to the sides of the legs (Figure 5-119).

You can use the same techniques on these two cavities that you used on the back of the hip: the thumb, the second and middle fingers, or the base of the palm (Figure 5-120). Press and rub in a circle. When you massage these cavities, start from the top one and move down to the bottom one. Again, do not use too much power, or you will cause tension.

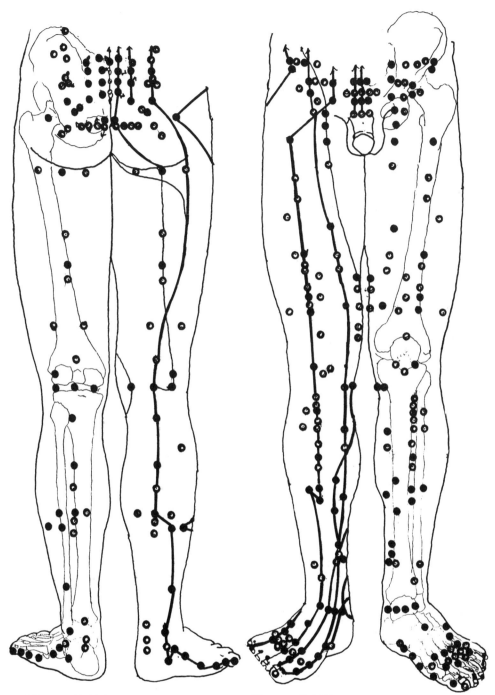

Figure 5-114.
Primary Qi channels and
acupuncture cavities on the leg
(back view).

Figure 5-115.
Primary Qi channels and
acupuncture cavities on the leg
(front view).

In order to lead the Qi further downward, another cavity called
Fengshi on the side of the thigh is also stimulated right after the
above two cavities. We will discuss this cavity later.

Figure 5-116. Primary Qi channels and acupuncture cavities on the leg (side view).

3.   Huiyin (Co-1):

The Huiyin (Meeting Yin) is located in the perineum midway between the genitals and the anus (Figure 5-121). In Chinese medicine and Qigong, the Huiyin is considered one of the most important cavities. It is the junction of many vessels, including the Conception, Governing, Thrusting, and Yin Heel Vessels.

Figure 5-117. The Zhongkong, Baihuanshu, Zhibian, Yinmen, Weizhong, and Chengshan cavities.

Remember, according to Chinese medicine, vessels are like reservoirs which regulate the Qi circulating in the twelve channels.

Stimulating the Huiyin cavity will improve the exchange of Qi among the vessels. According to Marrow/Brain Washing Qigong, holding up this area or pressing it correctly will lead Qi from the lower body upward through the Thrusting Vessel to nourish the marrow in the spine and also the brain. Experience in massage has shown that through stimulating this cavity, the Qi converted from the Pre-essence (hormone) which is produced by the testicles can be led downward to fill up the Qi in the Yin Heel Vessel. The Qi condition of this vessel is crucial for your leg strength. If you would like to know more about this subject, please refer to "Muscle/Tendon Changing and Marrow/Brain Washing Chi Kung" published by YMAA.

When you massage this gate, spread your partner's legs a comfortable distance apart. Press gently on the Huiyin cavity with your middle finger and circle around. If you use your right hand, circling clockwise will lead Qi upward to the brain, and counterclockwise will

Figure 5-118.

Figure 5-119 The Jiankua, Huantiao, and Fengshi cavities.

lead Qi downward to the legs (Figure 5-122). Frequently, the Xuehai cavity is massaged at the same time; this will be discussed later.

4.   Yinmen (B-51), Weizhong (B-54), and Chengshan (B-57):

Yinmen (Door of Abundance) is located in the middle of the back of the thigh, Weizhong (Commission the Middle) is right behind the knee, and Chengshan (Support the Mountain) is on the back of the calf (Figure 5-117). All of these gates belong to the Urine Bladder Qi channel. If you massage these three cavities right after you have loosened up the hip, you will be able to lead the Qi very quickly to the feet.

Because of the thick layer of muscle over Yinmen, the best way to massage it is to use a thumb, with the other thumb on top of it for support (Figure 5-123), though some people use the elbow or the bottom of the feet.

Figure 5-120.

Figure 5-121 The Huiyin cavity.

Figure 5-123.

Figure 5-122.

When you massage Weizhong and Chengshan, you can simply use the thumb or the second and middle fingers to rub the cavity (Figure 5-124). Again, it is common practice when working on these cavities to massage the Yongquan cavity at the same time to lead the Qi to the bottom of the feet.

5.   Fengshi (GB-31):
Fengshi (Wind's Market) is located in the center of the outside of the thigh (Figure 5-119). If you stimulate this cavity right after you have stimulated Jiankua and Huantiao on the side of the hip,

Figure 5-124.   Figure 5-125.

you will be able to lead Qi from the waist downward to the legs
very easily.

When you stimulate this cavity, you may use a thumb or the
base of a palm to press in firmly and then vibrate (Figure 5-125).
Frequently, the Jiexi cavity on the ankle will also be pressed to build
up the connection. Jiexi will be discussed below.

6.   Xuehai (Sp-10) and Sanyinjiao (Sp-6):

Xuehai (Sea of Blood) is located on the inner side of the thigh
near the knee. Sanyinjiao (Three Yin Junction) is located on the
lower inner section of the calf (Figure 5-126). When these cavities
are pressed and stimulated, the Qi circulating in the inner side of
the leg can be led downward.

When you massage these cavities, simply use the thumb to
press in firmly and then vibrate (Figure 5-127).

7.   Tiaokou (S-38) and Jiexi (S-41):

Tiaokou (Line's Opening) is located half-way down the chin, and
Jiexi (Release Stream) is located in the middle of the crease in the
front of the ankle (Figure 5-126). They both belong to the stomach
channel. When Tiaokou and Jiexi are pressed and stimulated, the
Qi on the front of the thigh can be led downward.

When you massage these two cavities, you may use a thumb or
the second and middle fingers to press in firmly and rub around
(Figure 5-128).

8.   Yongquan (K-1):

Younquan (Gushing Spring) is located on the sole of the foot, one
third of the way from the base of the second toe to the heel. It is the
final point on the kidney channel. It is an important Qi gate which
can regulate the Qi in the kidneys. Like the Laogong cavity in the
hand, stimulating this cavity will lead Qi from the torso downward
to the bottoms of the feet and spread it out there.

Figure 5-126. The Xuehai, Sanyinjiao, Tiaokou, and Jiexi cavities.

Figure 5-127.

Figure 5-128.

When you massage Yongquan, you can use a thumb to press in and circle firmly. When you use your right hand to circle clockwise on the right foot, you are nourishing the kidneys (Figure 5-129).

Figure 5-130.

Figure 5-129.

However, if you use your right hand to circle clockwise on the left foot, you will release Qi.

Massaging the Back of the Thighs and Legs:

Before you massage the legs, first cover your partner's body with a blanket or towel to keep them warm. After a massage, the pores in the skin are wide open, and it it easy to catch a cold.

Step #1:

First run your hands lightly over your partner's skin from their lower back to the bottom of their feet (Figure 5-130). Repeat several times. Next, repeat the same process on the sides of the waist, moving down along the sides of the legs to the bottom of the feet. Finally, do the same thing from the sacrum down the insides of the legs to the bottom of the feet. This will help your partner to relax, and also bring their mind back to their legs, which will help to lead the Qi there.

Step #2:

Next, massage and open the gates on the buttocks and upper legs. Before you do this, however, you should massage the lower back to loosen up the lower spine and the trunk muscles in the lower back.

Then, massage and stimulate the gates on the back of the hips (Zhongkong, Zhibian, and Yinmen) and the back of the knees and calves (Weizhong, and Chengshan). Finally massage the Yongquan on the bottom of the feet (Figure 5-131).

After you have opened up the back of the thighs and calves, stimulate and massage the gates on the outsides of the thighs and calves. These gates include Jiankua and Huantiao on the thigh, and Fengshi on the side of the thigh. After this, use your palm to push

Figure 5-131.   Figure 5-132.

downward gently from the side of the thigh to the foot (Figure 5-132), and finally massage the Yongquan cavity.

Next, stimulate and massage the gates on the inside of the legs. First massage Huiyin, and then Xuehai, Sanyinjiao, and finally Yongquan. Again, use your hands to brush downward on the inside of the thighs to the bottoms of the feet.

Finally, stimulate and massage the cavities on the front of the calf: Tiaokou, Jiexi, and Yongquan. When you massage these gates, bend your partner's leg to make it easier for you.

Step #3:

After you have stimulated and massaged the gates, you want to bring the accumulated Qi and blood to the surface. In order to do this, you first use the base or the edge of your palm to massage the lower back and sacrum for a few minutes. Next, use the base of your palms to press on the hips and then circle (Figure 5-133). If the circle moves up near the center and then to the sides, you are spreading the Qi and blood to the sides. This motion will also lead the Qi and blood upward. Therefore, circling in this direction is good for nourishing but not for releasing. However, if you circle in the other direction, you will lead the Qi and blood down. This will release the Qi and relax your partner. When you massage the hips, first do the entire back of the hips from the top to the bottom, and then the outsides of the hips, again from the top to the bottom.

Finally, grab the muscles on the back of the hips with your fingers and rub them (Figure 5-134). Remember, when you massage you do not want to cause any pain or uneasiness in your partner, since this will cause tension and hinder the massage.

If you have weak hands, you may use your knees (Figure 5-135) or foot to press the hip and then circle around. Your knees and feet can generate much more power than your hands, so you must be very careful when you use them.

Figure 5-133.

Figure 5-134.

Figure 5-135.

Figure 5-136.

Step #4:

After finishing the hips, raise the foot up to relax the thigh and calf muscles for an easier massage. Next, press down firmly with the base of your palm and then release on the back of the thighs from the top to the knees (Figure 5-136). If you find that you cannot generate enough penetrating power with one hand, you may use two hands (Figure 5-137). Repeat several times.

Next, use the base of both palms to press inward and circle evenly on the sides of the thighs downward to the knees (Figure 5-138). Repeat several times. When you do this, pay attention to the inside of the thighs. The inside of the thigh is tender and can be injured easily if you use power incorrectly. Also be careful that you do not rub the skin.

Figure 5-137.

Figure 5-138.

Figure 5-139.

Figure 5-140.

Next, grab the back of the thigh muscles with you fingers and rub from the top of the thigh to the knee (Figure 5-139). In order to prevent injuring the inside of the thighs, keep your thumbs on the outside and the other four fingers on the inside of the thighs. Repeat the entire process several times.

Next, use the sides of your palms to gently hit the backs and sides of the hips and thighs from the hips down to the knees (Figure 5-140). This will bring the accumulated Qi and blood to the surface. Repeat the procedure several times.

If your hands are too weak to massage the thigh muscles, you may use one or both feet instead (Figure 5-141). When you use the feet to

Figure 5-141.

Figure 5-142.

Figure 5-143

Figure 5-144.

massage, your foot should be as relaxed as possible. Simply place your foot on the thigh, and generate the motion with your knee or hip.

After you have completed this massage, brush downward several times with your hands on the backs, insides, and outsides of the hips and thighs from the hips to the knees (Figure 5-142).

Step #5:

Next, massage the calves. When you massage the calf, you may again keep your partner's feet in the raised position to relax the calf muscles. You may also place your partner's foot on your chest while you are massaging the calf.

Again, the inside of the calf is tender and can be injured easily if you are not careful. Grab the muscles on the back and sides of the

Figure 5-145.

Figure 5-146.

Figure 5-147.

Figure 5-148.

calf and rub downward from the knee to the ankle (Figure 5-143). Alternatively, you may also use the side of a palm to press and rub from the knee to the ankle (Figure 5-144).

Next, use both palms to press in gently and rub around from the knee to the ankle (Figure 5-145). Repeat the process several times.

Step #6:

Next, massage the ankle and foot. First, gently rub the skin on the ankle and foot for a few minutes (Figure 5-146). Then, hold the lower calf firmly but gently with one hand, and move the foot in a circle (Figure 5-147). Circle slowly and smoothly about twenty times in each direction.

Figure 5-149.   Figure 5-150.

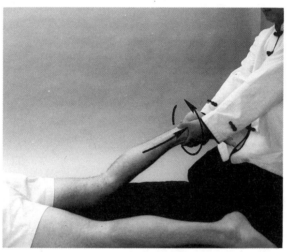

Figure 5-151.

Massage the ankle area with your fingers or the edge of your palm (Figure 5-148). Then press inward gently with your thumb and massage the entire ankle joint (Figure 5-149).

Next, use a thumb to massage the entire foot, especially the bottom of the foot, from the ankle to the toes (Figure 5-150). Repeat several times. Finally, grab every toe with your thumb and second finger and gently pull several times. You do not need to pop the joints.

Step #7:

After finishing the above massage, grab the foot or the lower section of the calf with both hands and lift up slightly. Pull gently and move the whole leg in a circle (Figure 5-151). Again, brush the entire leg from the hip downward to the bottom of the foot a few times to complete the leg massage.

Figure 5-152. Superficial anatomical structure of the posterior aspect of the arm.

During the course of the leg massage, you may repeatedly massage the gates whenever you are in the area; this will keep them open as you massage.

2. Massaging the Back of the Upper Arms, Forearms, and Hands:

Before massaging the arms, you should cover your partner's legs with a towel or blanket to keep them warm. However, this may not be needed if the room is warm enough.

Anatomical Structure of the Arm and Its Circulatory Systems:

Just beneath the skin on the back of the arm is muscle, some nerves extending from the shoulder down to the hand, and some veins on the back and inside of the arm (Figure 5-152).

Once all the muscles are removed, you can see the main nerve and artery coming down from the shoulder to the hand (Figure 5-153). You can also see some of the arteries and nerves extending from under the shoulder blade to the top of the shoulder.

Finally, you can see the front and the back of the hands (Figures 5-154 and 5-155). You can see in these two pictures that most of the

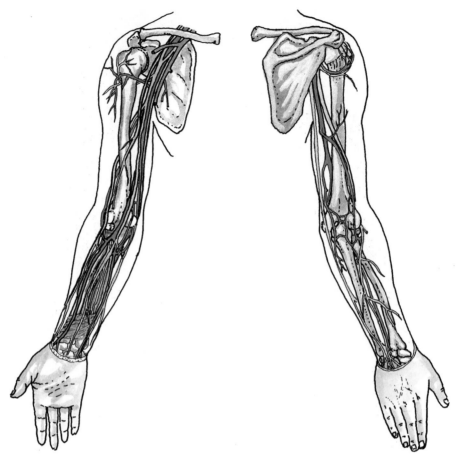

Figure 5-153. Deep anatomical structure of the posterior aspect of the arm.

Figure 5-154. Anatomical structure of the posterior aspect of the hand (front view).

Figure 5-155. Deep anatomical structure of the posterior aspect of the arm (back view).

blood circulatory system and the nerves are hidden in the gaps between the bones of the palm.

Theory:

After you have finished the legs, massage the arms to complete the massage of the back of the body. Like the legs, there are six primary Qi channels connected to the arms. Because of these channels, the arms are important in general massage, although they are not considered quite as important as the legs. This is because the muscles in the arms are not as large as those in the legs, and so there is less accumulation of Qi and blood in the arms, and it is more easily removed. In Tui Na massage, however, the arms are the most important area to massage for healing.

Like the legs, there are three Yin channels on the inside and three Yang channels on the outside of the arm. Therefore, the inside of the arm is more tender than the outside, and you should be gentler and more careful with your power.

The basic idea of arm massage is to lead the Qi accumulated in the upper body to the hands and finally release it from the body. We will next introduce the important gates on the back of the upper arm, forearm, and the hand, and then go on to discuss massage techniques. But first, please review the Qi circulatory system of the arms (Figure 5-156).

Gates:

1.   Jianliao (TB-14) and Jianyu (LI-15):

Jianliao (Shoulder Seam) and Jianyu (Shoulder Bone) are located in the shoulder area (Figure 5-157). When these two cavities are massaged and stimulated, Qi in the upper body can be led to the upper arms.

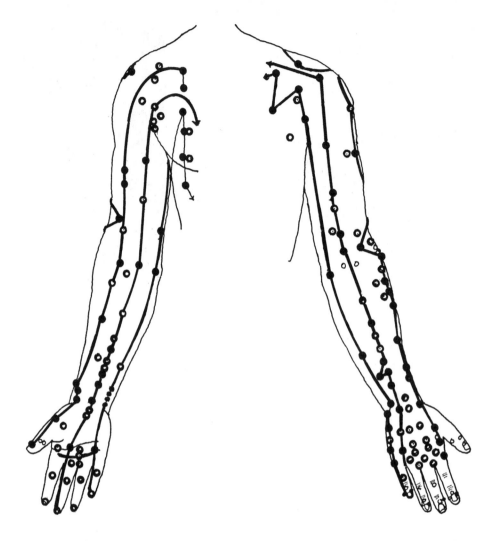

Figure 5-156. Primary Qi channels and acupuncture cavities on the arms.

To massage these two gates, you may use your thumb, second, or the middle finger to press on the cavity. If you are using the right hand on the right shoulder, you should circle in a counterclockwise direction (Figure 5-158). Naturally, if you are using the left hand on the left shoulder, you should circle in a clockwise direction.

2. Naohui (TB-13) and Binao (LI-14):

Naohui (Shoulder's Meeting) and Binao (Arm and Scapula) are located on the outside of the upper arm (Figures 5-157 and 5-159). When these two cavities are massaged and stimulated, the Qi in the shoulders can be led to the arms.

To massage these two gates, you may use the thumb, the second and the middle fingers, or the middle finger to press on the cavity and then rub in a counterclockwise circle if you are using your right hand (Figure 5-160), or clockwise if you are using your left hand.

Jianliao (TB-14)

Jianyu (LI-15)

Binao (LI-14)

Quchi (LI-11)

Hegu (LI-4)

Figure 5-157. The Jianyu, Jianliao, Biano, Quchi, and Hegu cavities.

Figure 5-158.

Naohui (TB-13)

Sidu (TB-9)

Figure 5-159. The Naohui and Sidu cavities.

Figure 5-160.

Chize (L-5)

Kongzui (L-6)

Figure 5-161. The Chize and Kongzui cavities.

3. Quchi (LI-11) and Chize (L-5):

Quchi (Crooked Pool) and Chize (Cubit Marsh) are located near the elbow (Figures 5-157 and 5-161). When they are massaged and stimulated, Qi in the upper arm can be led downward to the elbow.

To massage these two gates, you may use your thumb or the middle finger to press on the cavity and then rub in a counterclockwise circle if you are using your right hand. If you are using your left hand, you should circle in a clockwise direction (Figure 5-162).

4. Kongzui (L-6) and Sidu (TB-9):

Kongzui (Opening Maximum) is located on the inside of the forearm, while Sidu (Four Ditch) is located on the outside (Figures 5-159 and 5-161). When they are massaged and stimulated, Qi in the upper arm can be led downward to the forearm.

To massage these two gates, you may use your thumb or middle finger to press on the cavity and rub in a counterclockwise circle if you are using your right hand, and clockwise if you are using your left hand (Figure 5-163).

5. Hegu (LI-4):

Hegu (Adjoining Valleys) is located on the base of the thumb

Figure 5-162.

Figure 5-163.

Figure 5-164.

Laogong (P-8)

Figure 5-165. The Laogong cavity.

and the second finger (Figure 5-157). When this cavity is massaged and stimulated, Qi in the back of the arm can be led to the hand.

To massage these two gates, you may use your thumb to press on the cavity and then rub in a counterclockwise direction if you are using your right hand (Figure 5-164), and in a clockwise direction if you are using your left hand.

6. Laogong (P-8):

Laogong (Labor's Palace) is located in the center of the palm (Figure 5-165). The exact point is where the tip of the middle finger touches the palm. The two Laogong cavities are two of the four main gates on the limbs from which Qi inside the body can communicate with the Qi outside of the body. When the Laogong is massaged and stimulated, Qi can be led to the palms.

To massage Laogong, you may use your right thumb to press on the cavity and rub in a counterclockwise direction (Figure 5-166). If

Figure 5-166.   Figure 5-167.

you circle in the other direction, you will be nourishing the Qi instead of releasing it.

Massaging the Back of the Upper Arms, Forearms, and Hands:
Step #1:

First, brush your hands lightly over your partner's skin from their shoulders to their hands (Figure 5-167). Repeat several times. This will help them relax, and also bring their mind to their arms, which will bring a significant amount of Qi from their upper body to the arms.

Next, place your partner's arm behind their back and use both your hands to raise the shoulder gently and move it in a circle (Figure 5-168). When you circle the right arm, move it in a clockwise direction, and when you circle the left arm move it in a counterclockwise direction. This circular motion can relax the entire shoulder and can also help your partner to lead Qi to the arm.

Step #2:

Next, massage and open the gates on the shoulders and arms. Before you do this, you should massage the upper back again and relax the upper body. Then again stimulate the Jianjing cavity located between the neck and the shoulder (Figure 5-169). You should also massage the Tianzong cavity in the center of the shoulder blade (Figure 5-170).

After you have loosened up the upper body and the shoulders, use the massage techniques introduced earlier to massage and stimulate all of the gates located on the shoulders and arms. You should start from the shoulder and move down to the hand. Repeat the process several times.

Step #3:

Next, use the base of your palms to sandwich the arm, gently squeezing and rubbing it around (Figure 5-171). Start at the shoulder and move down to the forearm. Repeat several times.

Figure 5-168.

Figure 5-169.

Figure 5-170.

Figure 5-171.

Step #4:
Next, use your thumb and fingers to grab and rub the muscles from the shoulders to the forearms (Figure 5-172). Repeat several times.

Step #5:
Next, gently slap the entire arm from the shoulder to the forearm (Figure 5-173). This will lead the Qi underneath to the surface of the skin. Finally, use a hand to brush from the shoulder to the forearm several times.

Figure 5-172.

Figure 5-173.

Figure 5-174.

Figure 5-175.

Step #6:

Finally, hold your partner's hand with one hand and the forearm with the other and move the wrist around several times (Figure 5-174). Then, use a thumb to rub the entire hand from the wrist down to every fingertip (Figure 5-175). Next, grab the forearm with both hands and gently pull the entire arm once (Figure 5-176), and then grab each finger and pull gently (Figure 5-177). When you pull the fingers, you do not have to pop the joints.

During the course of the arm massage, you may repeatedly massage the gates whenever you are in the area. This will keep them open.

Figure 5-176.   Figure 5-177.

5-6. Massaging the Chest and Abdomen
Anatomical Structure of the Front of the Body and Its Circulatory Systems:

Beneath the skin and the layer of fat on the front of the body, we first see the muscles, and many nerves spreading out from underneath the muscles (Figure 5-178). In addition, there are many veins distributed over the entire area. Other than on the chest near the armpits, there is not too much thick muscle on the front of the body. Beneath the muscles on the ribs, there are two sets of large trunk muscles running from the chest down to the groin area.

With all of the muscles removed, you can see some of the internal organs. The lungs and the heart are behind the ribs. Under the solar plexus is the stomach. On the left of the stomach (looking from the front) is the liver, and behind the liver is the gall bladder; while on the right is the spleen. Under these organs are the large and small intestines as well as, in women, the uterus and ovaries, and finally, below the intestines is the urinary bladder (Figure 5-179).

Theory:

Neither China nor the West place much emphasis upon massaging the front of the body. This is due primarily to the fact that most people feel more tension in the back of their bodies, but also because most people are more ticklish in the front, and they are more likely to become uneasy and tense if improper massaging techniques are employed. In addition, the sexual areas are in the front of the body, and massaging near them would make many people feel uncomfortable, especially in the ancient, conservative societies. For these reasons, more massage techniques have been developed for the back than for the front of the body.

Figure 5-178. Superficial anatomical structure of the anterior aspect of
the trunk.

Figure 5-179. Deep anatomical structure
of the anterior aspect of the
trunk.

From the purely physical point of view, the trunk muscles in the
back are usually more tense when a person is tired or fatigued.
Since the center of the body's nervous system is in the spine, massaging the back can easily bring the entire body into a relaxed state.
However, from the point of view of Chinese medicine and Qigong,
massaging the front of the body is at least as important as massaging the back.

First, according to Chinese medicine, the Conception Vessel
runs down the center of the front of the body. This is a Yin vessel,
and it is responsible for regulating the Qi level in the six Yin
primary Qi channels. In order for it to do this effectively, the center
of the front of the body must be relaxed.

Second, most of the internal organs are located in the front of the body, and in giving a massage you reach them through the front of the body. The internal organs are right behind the front trunk muscles. We already know that problems in the internal organs are the cause of most illnesses. The internal organs are like machines in the production line of life. Whenever one of them malfunctions, life can be threatened. Because of this, maintaining smooth Qi circulation in and among the internal organs is a very important part of Chinese Qigong massage. The way to improve Qi circulation in the internal organs is to relax the muscles which surround them. This is why the goal of massaging the front of the body in Chinese Qigong massage is to relax the front trunk muscles.

Furthermore, according to Chinese medicine and Qigong, the lower abdomen is the site of the Lower Dan Tian, which is the residence of Original Qi. Original Qi is the source of life energy, so increasing the flow of this Qi from its residence is an important part of massage.

Normally, after you have finished massaging the back and start massaging the front of the body, you again begin at the head and lead the Qi downward to the chest area. After massaging the chest and abdomen, you continue on to the front of the legs to lead the Qi further downward. Finish your massage with the arms. In order to know the Qi gates on the front of the body, you need to be familiar with the Qi circulatory system. Figure 5-180 shows the Governing Vessel and all of the primary channels located on the front of the body. Next, we will introduce the gates on the front of the body, and then follow this discussion with some massage techniques.

Gates:
1. Tiantu (Co-22):
Tiantu (Heaven's Prominence) is located on the base of the throat and is the junction of the neck and the chest (Figure 5-181). In acupuncture, the function of this cavity is to facilitate and regulate the movement of lung Qi in order to cool the throat and to clear the voice. When this gate is relaxed and wide open, the Qi communication between the throat and the chest can be smooth.

When you massage this gate, you must be very gentle. Start from the side of the gate and follow the bone, using the fingers of both hands to brush toward the Tiantu cavity a few times (Figure 5-182). Next, use your thumb or the second and third fingers to rub the cavity very gently with a circular motion (Figure 5-183). Circle in a counterclockwise direction and lead the Qi downward to the chest.

2. Shufu (K-27) and Qihu (S-13):
Shufu (Hollow Residence) and Qihu (Qi's Household) are located above the nipples (Figure 5-181). Shufu belongs to the kidney channel. The kidneys have a primary role in water metabolism and controlling the body's liquids. When the Shufu cavity is massaged and stimulated, the water in the body can be led upward to the

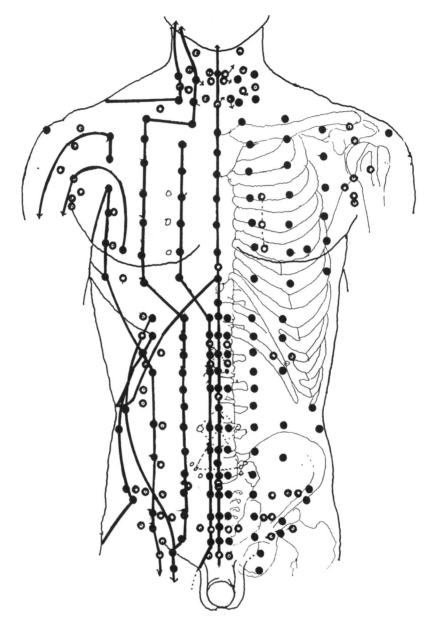

Figure 5-180. Primary Qi channels and acupuncture cavities on the front of the body.

lungs. In Chinese medicine, this cavity is related to bronchitis, asthma, chest pain, vomiting, and abdominal distension.

When Qihu is massaged and stimulated, the Qi accumulated in the center of the lungs can be spread to the sides of the lungs, which will relax the chest. In addition, massaging Qihu will lead the Qi accumulated in the neck downward to the chest. In Chinese medicine, Qihu is related to such illnesses as bronchitis, asthma, hiccups, and intercostal neuralgia

When you massage these two cavities, rub in a circle with your second and middle fingers. Circle to the center and then up, and finally to the sides of the chest and out the arms (Figure 5-184).

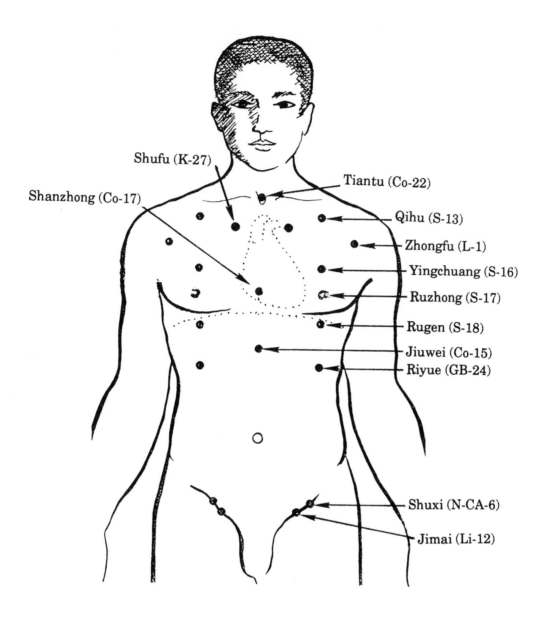

Figure 5-181. The Tiantu, Qihu, Shufu, Zhongfu, Yinchuang, Shanzhong, Ruzhong, Rugen, Jiuwei, Riyue, Shuxi, and Jimai cavities.

3. Zhongfu (L-1):

Zhongfu (Central Residence) is located in the upper chest near the shoulder joint (Figure 5-181). According to Chinese medicine, this cavity is connected to the throat area, as well as to the lungs and stomach. This cavity is the junction of the throat and upper chest with the arms. Therefore, massage will lead the Qi accumulated on the front of the neck and upper chest out to the shoulders and finally to the hands, where it can be dissipated. In Chinese medicine, this cavity is related to coughing and wheezing, coughing blood and pus, throat blockage, nasal congestion, excessive sweating, tumors and nodular growths on the neck.

Figure 5-182.

Figure 5-183.

Figure 5-184.

Figure 5-185.

When you massage this cavity, simply use the second and middle fingers to press in and circle a few times, and then brush with your hands out to the arms (Figure 5-185). When you massage, circle toward the center and then upward and finally to the side. This will lead the Qi to the arms.

4. Shanzhong (Co-17):

Shanzhong (Penetrating Odor) is located directly between the nipples (Figure 5-181). When Shanzhong is massaged correctly, the Qi accumulated in the center of the chest can be spread outward.

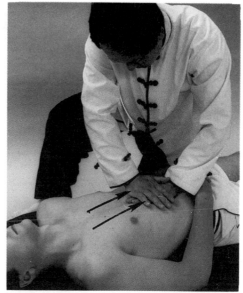

Figure 5-186.   Figure 5-187.

This can significantly regulate the Fire Qi which has accumulated in the solar plexus (Middle Dan Tian). This will release pressure and tension in the front of the body. In Chinese medicine, treating this cavity can regulate and suppress rebellious Qi, and expand the chest to benefit the diaphragm.

To massage this cavity, use the base of a palm to gently press the cavity and rub in a circle a few times, then lead the Qi to the sides and away from the solar plexus (Figure 5-186). Use your right hand to circle clockwise, then spread to the side of the chest a few times, and then circle with your left hand in a counterclockwise direction the same number of times. Finally, use the palms to push downward to the abdominal area (Figure 5-187). In order to avoid leading Qi to the solar plexus, do not stop your pushing at the solar plexus area.

5.   Jiuwei (Co-15):

Jiuwei (Wild Pigeon's Tail) is called the solar plexus in the West, and the Middle Dan Tian in Chinese Qigong. The Middle Dan Tian is the residence of Fire Qi or Post-birth Qi, which is converted from air and food. Physically, this place is the junction between the lungs and the stomach, which is beneath the diaphragm. Whenever too much Qi accumulates in this area, you will feel uncomfortable and experience tension or heartburn in your chest. Because of the excess Yang, you will feel tired. One of the practices of Chinese Qigong is to lead the Qi accumulated here downward to the Lower Dan Tian. In Chinese medicine, this cavity is related to such illnesses as angina pectoris, seizures, hiccups, mental illness, and asthma.

Massaging Jiuwei correctly will loosen the area so that the Qi can be moved easily and spread either to the sides or downward to the lower body. The method of massaging this cavity is very simple.

Figure 5-188.   Figure 5-189.

Gently rub the cavity in a clockwise circular motion with the base of your right palm, and then lead the Qi to the side (Figure 5-188). Repeat several times. Then change to the left hand and repeat the same massage, only now use a counterclockwise motion and lead the Qi down. Finally, use the palms to push downward to the abdomen (Figure 5-189).

6.   Yingchuang (S-16), Ruzhong (S-17), and Rugen (S-18):

     Yingchuang (Breast's Window), Ruzhong (Middle of Breast), and Rugen (Breast's Root) are located above the nipple, in the middle of the nipple, and under the nipple (Figure 5-181). These three cavities are usually treated as one in Qigong massage. They are related to bronchitis, mastitis, asthma, intercostal neuralgia, intestinal noises and diarrhea.

     Beneath these cavities is a large section of muscle which extends out to the front of the shoulder. When these muscles are relaxed, the Qi can be led easily to the sides of the chest and also to the front of the shoulder. When you massage these three cavities, first place your index, middle, and ring fingers on all three cavities at the same time, and move your fingers in circles (Figure 5-190). In order to avoid leading Qi toward the solar plexus, you should lead the Qi to the sides of the chest and shoulders.

7.   Riyue (GB-24):

     Riyue (Sun Moon) is located below the ribs in front of the liver and spleen (Figure 5-181). When there is an abnormal Qi condition in the liver and spleen, these two cavities may be tense, which will cause tension in the stomach and abdomen. In Qigong massage, in order to relax the internal organs below the diaphragm you need to

Figure 5-190.   Figure 5-191.

relax these cavities. In Chinese medicine, this cavity is related to intercostal neuralgia, cholecystitis, acute and chronic hepatitis, peptic ulcer, and hiccups.

To massage these cavities, use the base of your palms to gently press the cavities and rub in a circle a few times, and then lead the motion to the center and move downward (Figure 5-191). When you massage, the right hand should circle counterclockwise and the left hand clockwise. You should also massage in the opposite direction and follow the ribs to lead the Qi to the sides (Figure 5-192).

8. Shuxi (N-CA-6) and Jimai (Li-12):

Shuxi (Mouse Path) and Jimai (Urgent Pulse) are located in the crease between the thigh and abdomen (Figure 5-181). These two cavities are the junctions of the Qi circulation from the body to the legs in the front of the body. In Chinese medicine, Shuxi is related to tuberculosis of the inguinal lymph glands, and weakness of leg adductors. Jimai is related to prolapsed uterus, pain of hernia, and pain in the penis.

When you massage these two cavities, simply use the edge of your palm to press in and circle (Figure 5-193) while raising your partner's thigh to relax the area.

Massaging the Chest and Abdomen:
Step #1:

First, use your hands to lightly and slowly brush from the face down over the chest, and finally down to the legs and the bottoms of the feet (Figure 5-194). Repeat five times. Then repeat the same process again, now brushing from the face, over the shoulders and finally down to the hands (Figure 5-195). Repeat five times.

Figure 5-192.

Figure 5-193.

Figure 5-194.

Figure 5-195.

Step #2:

Next, gently stimulate and massage the gates discussed above. Massage the top gates first, and move downward to the abdomen. This will make it easier for the Qi and blood to circulate. Frequently your partner will be ticklish and will tense up. If this happens, change your techniques so that they can relax again. For example, if you started using your fingers, you may switch to using your palms.

Step #3:

Next, massage the centerline on the front of the body, leading the Qi downward. To do this, stroke downward with both hands from the back of the neck to the upper chest, and then follow the centerline downward to the abdomen (Figure 5-196). Repeat five times.

Figure 5-196.

Figure 5-197.

Figure 5-198.

Figure 5-199.

Then use both hands to gently press the center of the chest from the upper chest to the solar plexus (Figure 5-197).

Step #4:

Use the second and middle fingers of both hands to gently massage the areas above the nipples and under the shoulders for one minute. If your partner is ticklish, switch to your palms (Figure 5-198). This will lead the kidney Qi and water upward to moisten the lungs.

Next, place both palms on the center of the upper chest and push the palms to the sides of the upper chest (Figure 5-199). When

Figure 5-200.   Figure 5-201.

you do this, you should push along the ribs with your fingers between the ribs. Again, if your partner is ticklish, use your palms instead. This will spread the Qi and moisture which were led upward to the sides of the lungs. Repeat five times.

Finally, repeat the same process, however, start from the solar plexus area and move to the sides from of the chest (Figure 5-200). Repeat five times.

Step #5:

Using the base or the edge of both palms, rub from the top of the chest to the diaphragm area with a circular motion (Figure 5-201). Repeat five times. The direction of the circle is very important. When your right hand is circling counterclockwise while your left hand is circling clockwise, you are leading the Qi downward, which will cool down the body. If you reverse the direction, you are leading the Qi upward. This is not desirable in general massage, because it can lead the Qi to the head and make the body too Yang.

Step #6:

Next, use your thumb and fingers to grab and rub the tendons in the front of the armpits (Figure 5-202). Continue the grabbing and rubbing downward to the area of the nipples, and then use your palm to smooth and lead Qi down from the armpit (Figure 5-203). Repeat the same procedure about five times. If your partner is very ticklish, simply use your palms to rub in circles downward (Figure 5-204).

Step #7:

After you have finished the chest massage, move downward to massage the stomach, abdomen, and waist. First, place both hands on your partner's stomach and circle gently in a clockwise direction

Figure 5-202.

Figure 5-203.

Figure 5-204.

Figure 5-205.

(Figure 5-205). Circle about ten to twenty times. While circling your hands, your mind should be very calm and relaxed, and you should be paying attention to where the stomach is located inside the body. Then repeat the same process on the abdomen.

Step #8:

Place your hands on both sides of the centerline at the level of your partner's diaphragm. Ask your partner to inhale and then exhale deeply. While they are exhaling, brush both hands downward to the groin area (Figure 5-206).

Figure 5-206.   Figure 5-207.

Then bend one of your partner's legs. With one hand holding the leg in place, massage the area around the front of the hip joint (Figure 5-207). After rubbing in a circle a few times, stroke your hand to the thigh. Repeat a few times. Repeat the same process on the other side.

Finally, spread your partner's legs a comfortable distance apart, and use your middle finger to gently massage the Huiyin cavity (Figure 5-208). As mentioned before, this cavity is very important in Chinese Qigong practice.

Step #9:

The last step in massaging the front of the body is the waist area. First, use both hands to massage the muscles on the sides of the waist a few times (Figure 5-209). Then gently raise up the waist area and release it a couple of times (Figure 5-210). Finally, brush your hands from the waist to the front of the legs a few times (Figure 5-211).

5-7. Massaging the Front of the Limbs

We have already discussed the basic theory of massage when we discussed the massage of the back of the arms and legs, and we have introduced the gates on the back and sides of the thighs, upper arms, calves, feet, forearms, and hands. It is recommended that you go over the section about the massage of the back of the limbs before beginning this section.

In the previous section we discussed the structure of the arms and legs, now we will begin by introducing the gates of the thighs and upper arms. Next, we will discuss massage techniques for massaging the limbs when you partner is lying on his/her back.

Figure 5-208.

Figure 5-209.

Figure 5-211.

Figure 5-210.

Legs:
Gates on the Front of the Thigh:
1.   Futu (S-32):

Futu (Hidden Rabbit) is located on the lower section of the front of the thigh (Figure 5-212). When the Qi circulation in this cavity is stagnant, the lower limb can be paralyzed. Blockage of the Qi in this cavity can cause pain in the waist and the groin area. Futu is frequently used for treating arthritis in the knees.

When this cavity is stimulated properly, the Qi in the lower body can be led downward. To stimulate this cavity, the thumb is generally

Figure 5-212. The Xuehai and Futu cavities.

Figure 5-213.

Figure 5-214.

used to press down on the cavity and then vibrate (Figure 5-213). However, the elbow is sometimes used to generate a more penetrating power (Figure 5-214). Normally, right after stimulation, the side or the base of the palm is used to rub downward to the knee.

Figure 5-216.

Figure 5-215.

2. Xuehai (Sp-10):

This cavity was covered in the section on massage of the back of the leg.

Techniques
Legs:
Step #1:

First, hold one knee with both hands and rotate the leg in the hip joint about five times in both directions (Figure 5-215), and then repeat the same process for the other leg. This will loosen up the area of the hip joint.

Next, lightly brush downward with your hands a few times from the hips to the bottom of the feet, covering the front and both sides of the legs (Figure 5-216). This will relax the leg muscles.

Step #2:

Starting at the hip area, rub with the base of your palms from the hip joints down to the knees on the front of the thighs (Figure 5-217). There are three main paths on the front of the thighs: the center and the two sides.

Next, grab and rub the muscles on the top of the thighs, moving from the hips down to the knees (Figure 5-218). Then rub with the base or the edge of your palms from the hips down the outside of the thighs (Figure 5-219), and from the groin down the inside of the legs to the knees (Figure 5-220).

Step #3:

Use your thumb, index finger, and/or middle finger (whichever is easier and more convenient) to press and vibrate the gates in the

Figure 5-217.

Figure 5-218.

Figure 5-219.

Figure 5-220.

thighs (Figure 5-221). This will stimulate the cavities and enhance the Qi circulation in the primary channels. When you stimulate these cavities, start at the hips and work downward.

Step #4:
Use the edge of your palms to hit the front of the thighs gently from the top to the knee a few times (Figure 5-222). Repeat the same process for the external and internal sides. When you have finished, brush downward with your hands from the hips to the feet (Figure 5-223). Repeat several times.

Figure 5-221.

Figure 5-222.

Figure 5-223.

Figure 5-224.

Step #5:

Again massage the calves and feet. Since we have discussed them before, we will not cover them again. However, before you massage the feet, you should add an extra process: hold each ankle with both hands and move it in a circle a few times, and then gently pull the leg a few times (Figure 5-224).

Arms:
Gates on the Front of the Upper Arm:
1.   Jubi (N-UE-10):

Jubi (Raise Arm) is located on the front of the upper arm near the shoulder joint (Figure 5-225). When the Qi circulation in this cavity is blocked or stagnant, the arm will become numb.

Figure 5-225. The Jianneiling, Jubi, and Quze cavities.

To massage this cavity, simply rub the cavity with your thumb in a circular motion (Figure 5-226). Many people also use a thumb or index finger to press on the cavity and then release it a few times.

2. Jianneiling (M-UE-48):

Jianneiling (Shoulder's Inner Tomb) is also located on the front near the shoulder joint (Figure 5-225). Like Jubi, when the Qi circulation in this cavity is blocked or stagnant, the arm will become numb. This cavity and Jubi are frequently used in the treatment of arthritis in the shoulders.

To massage this cavity, simply rub the cavity with a circular motion with your thumb or index finger (Figure 5-227).

3. Quze (P-3):

Quze (Crooked Marsh) is located near the elbow joint (Figure 5-225). Its functions are opening the heart Qi, draining heat from the blood, and regulating the intestines.

When the Qi circulation is blocked or stagnant, chest pain can be experienced. This cavity is also known to be related to emotions

Figure 5-226.   Figure 5-227.

such as fright. In addition, it is significantly related to heat exhaustion, diarrhea with vomiting (acute gastroenteritis), fever, irritability, and fullness in the body.

To massage this cavity, use the thumb to press on the cavity and rub in little circles (Figure 5-228).

Massage of the Arms, Forearms, and Hands:
Step #1:

First, lightly brush your hands over your partner's skin from their shoulders to their hands (Figure 5-229). Repeat several times. This will help them relax, and also bring their mind to the arms, which will lead a significant amount of Qi from the upper body to the arms.

Step #2:

Massage and open the gates on the shoulders and arms. Before you do this, you should massage the upper chest again to relax the upper body. Then again stimulate the Jianjing cavity, which is located between the neck and the shoulder (Figure 5-230).

After you have loosened up the upper body and the shoulders, use the massage techniques introduced earlier to massage and stimulate all of the gates located on the shoulders and arms. You should start from the shoulders and move down to the hands. Repeat the same process several times.

Step #3:

Next, grab the muscles with your thumb and all four fingers and rub in a circular motion from the shoulder to the forearm (Figure 5-231). Repeat several times. Finally, repeat the massage procedures for the forearm and hands which were discussed earlier.

Figure 5-228.

Figure 5-229.

Figure 5-230.

Figure 5-231.

During the course of massaging the arms you may massage the gates again whenever you are near them; this will keep them open as you massage.

Chapter 6
General Self-Massage

6-1. General Concepts

Self-massage is a natural, human instinct to soothe the mind/spirit and ease discomfort in the body. There are many examples of this. If you accidentally get hit with a hard object, you naturally rub the hurt place to lessen the pain and also to keep a bruise from forming. When you sprain an ankle or injure any other joint, you automatically stroke the joint with your hands. Also, when an arm or leg has fallen asleep, you will sometimes hit it gently with a fist to restore feeling. And finally, when you feel discomfort in your stomach or any other internal organ, you rub it gently with your hand, and soon the discomfort goes away. All of these are examples of using self-massage to improve the Qi and blood circulation in an area where pain or discomfort is felt, in order to lessen the discomfort.

Now, let us consider some other examples. When your neck or back is stiff, what is your natural reaction? In the case of your neck, you will move your head in a circle or side to side to relax it. Similarly, when your back is stiff, you flex your back, twist it from side to side, or stretch it by bending forward. What do you do when you feel discomfort in the area of your solar plexus - or tension in any other internal organ - caused by being in an improper posture for a long time, such as sitting in front of a computer? Your natural reaction is to stand up and stretch your arms while taking a few deep breaths, and sometimes you will move your body around or move your waist in a circle a few times. All of these actions release tension and let you feel comfortable again.

If you understand these natural, human reactions, then you can easily understand what self-massage is. We can therefore define self-massage as "using the hands to rub the body, or using body movement, to release tension in the body or internal organs by improving the Qi and blood circulation."

The highest level of massage is Chinese Qigong massage, which uses Qi manipulation rather than purely physical massage.

However, this cannot be done unless you have had Qigong training. In Qi self-massage, the Qigong practitioner is able to use their mind to release the tension or pressure in tensed areas. He or she can also use the mind to circulate Qi in that area in order to speed up the healing process. The theory behind this is very simple. Your entire body (which includes both your Qi body and your physical body) is governed by your mind. Originally, we were able to use our minds to lead Qi to every part of the body to cause it to move. However, through the many years of "civilized" living we have gradually lost the instinct for this mind-body control, which most other animals still have. Through proper practice, we can regain this mind-body correspondence. In fact, this is the basic theory of all Chinese Qigong practice - returning to the natural way (Dao).

In this chapter, we will first review the goals of self-massage and also list the advantages and disadvantages of self-massage compared to massage by a partner. Next, in section 6-2, we will introduce self-massage using the hands. Then, in section 6-3, we will introduce two methods of internal organ self-massage: using the hands and using movement.

Goals of Self-Massage

Although many of the purposes of self-massage are obvious, from the viewpoint of Chinese Qigong its functions are both wider and more profound. In this section we would like to review these purposes so that you will have a clearer understanding of the "why" of this practice.

1. To remove any stagnation of Qi and blood and to increase their circulation. We have explained this goal already in our discussion of massage. One of the main goals of self-massage is improving the Qi and blood circulation in the whole body - especially the head, eyes, ears, and scalp.

2. To lessen pain and discomfort due to injury, and also to speed up the healing process. This refers to injuries where there is no break in the skin, such as bruises caused by being struck, and swollen joints caused by improper posture during sports or exercise. When this kind of injury occurs, blood cells accumulate at the site of the injury and create a bruise. In addition, the injury causes over stimulation of the area. This, in turn, results in the accumulation of a great amount of Qi, and a localized increase in temperature. These effects are all part of our body's natural, automatic reactions, and serve to keep out invading bacteria. However, the over stimulation of the area causes pain and discomfort. This can be reduced by quickly smoothing out the Qi and blood circulation. This will also insure that the cells receive the proper amount of fresh blood and Qi which they need to make repairs. Of course, you have to make sure that you do the massage very carefully. For example, if a bone has been cracked or broken, you must make sure that the massage does not interfere with the healing process. This will be discussed more extensively in the section in the next volume on Tui Na massage, which specializes in treating physical injuries.

3. To maintain and to improve smooth Qi and blood circulation in the internal organs. This is one of the main purposes of self-massage. When the internal organs fail, people get sick and even die. Therefore, keeping the internal organs healthy and functioning properly is one of the major subjects of Chinese Qigong. The key to doing this is maintaining the smooth circulation of Qi and blood. Self-massage accomplishes this in two ways: using the hands to massage the internal organs, and using body movement to exercise the internal organs. In fact, internal organ massage (Nei Zang An Mo) has proven to be very effective in treating almost every type of internal organ problem.

4. To help you understand your Qi body and physical body better. People usually get sick because of their unhealthy lifestyle and bad habits. It is very easy for the mind to ignore the body when it complains. In fact, most of the time our minds and bodies are acting independently, and they do not communicate and cooperate with each other smoothly and harmoniously. To be effective in self-massage, you must first learn to understand your body, and you must learn to use your mind to move your body in the most efficient way. Furthermore, you must learn to use your mind to feel the Qi in your body and to lead it. When your Qi body and your physical body are unified, they will be able to act together as one body.

5. To help you learn how to diagnose yourself. After you have unified your Qi and physical bodies, you will know yourself better, and you will be able to feel or even see any problem in your body. If you can feel or see a problem, then you will know how to correct it. Self-massage gradually teaches you how to see within your body and diagnose yourself.

6. To teach you how to massage others. Massage is done through feeling and mutual mental-correspondence between you and your partner. In Qigong An Mo, you merge with your partner so that you feel what they are feeling. Through physical touch and mutual Qi correspondence, the Qi is re-balanced. Self-massage teaches you how to regulate your mind and breathing, and also teaches you how to use your mind to lead the Qi to nourish your own body.

For example, when you feel uncomfortable somewhere in your body, you may massage the area either with your hands or with certain body movements. In order to make the massage effective, you must also use your mind to deeply relax the massaged area, which will allow the Qi to circulate smoothly and deeply. In addition, you can also use your mind to lead the Qi to the massaged area. Only when you combine both the external massage of your hands or body movements, and the internal massage of your concentrated mind, can the massage be truly effective. This means that when you practice self-massage, not only are you training the physical massage techniques, but, more importantly, you are also practicing how to use your mind to feel inside your body and make the massage more efficient. Once you have mastered the techniques of self-massage and are familiar with how Qi feels, then you will be able to communicate with other people's bodies with your mind and your feeling for Qi, and massage them effectively. Massaging yourself is the best way to gain experience before massaging others.

You can see that there are two sides to self-massage: the ability to sense what is going on inside and move the Qi there, and the physical techniques. The internal side is Yin and the external side is Yang. When the Yin participates, the external Yang massage can reach deep and be effective. Without the Yin, the massage will remain superficial.

Advantages and Disadvantages of Self-Massage
In this sub-section, we will summarize the advantages and the disadvantages of self-massage when compared to massage by a partner.

Advantages of Self-Massage:
1.   Self-massage gives you a better understanding of your Qi and physical bodies. It increases your sensitivity, and improves the communications between your Qi body and your physical body, which is the foundation of self-diagnosis. In Chinese Qigong, accurate self-diagnosis is one of the most important keys to regulating Qi disorders before any physical damage occurs. When you massage someone else, your attention is on their body, and you usually tend to ignore your own body. It is like the physician who constantly tells his patients how to prevent sickness, but gets sick himself because he fails to pay more attention to himself. Feeling inside yourself is the key to maintaining health.

2.   Self-massage improves your mind-body coordination. When someone else is massaging you, you have to coordinate your mind with their mind and techniques. Similarly, when you massage someone else, you have to have their full mental cooperation in order to be effective. This is difficult to achieve when you have just met, and aren't fully comfortable with each other yet. This problem does not arise when you massage yourself, and it is much easier for you to correct Qi irregularities in your own body. With self-massage, your mind can coordinate with and control the power of the techniques. This enables you to avoid the pain and bruises that sometimes occur in cavity press massage when the minds and feelings of the masseur and patient are not in communication.

3.   Self-massage is convenient. Since you do not need a partner, it can be done anytime and anyplace.

Disadvantages of Self-Massage:

1. A general, massage is more relaxing and more enjoyable when someone else massages you. When massage is used for relaxation and improving the general Qi and blood circulation, rather than for healing, concentrating your mind is not so important. When someone is massaging you, you can simply relax as much as possible and enjoy the experience. Self-massage is not as satisfying, because it is not possible to completely relax.

2. It is very easy to be lazy and let your emotional mind dominate you. Even though you know that you should massage yourself, it is very easy to skip the massage. However, if you have a regular time when someone else massages you, or you massage each other, it is much harder to break the pattern. Most people usually do not take self-massage seriously until they are really sick. They forget that regular self-massage is the best way to maintain their health. It is very easy to find excuses for not massaging oneself. A common one is when people have bruises, and they complain that massaging around a bruise can hurt. It is often hard for us to discipline ourselves and do what is best.

3. It is impossible to massage some parts of your own body. The spine is a vital part of both the Qi circulatory system and the nervous system, and it is very important to massage it. Unfortunately, the only way you can massage your own spine is through certain movements, and this is not as effective as using the hands. Other areas that are difficult to massage yourself are the shoulders, the back of the neck, and the back of the thighs.

4. When you massage yourself, you miss the opportunity to share your feelings with another person. Also, with mutual massage it is often easier to regulate and balance each other's Qi. One of the practices of Qigong is to obtain a better Qi balance through Qi communication with a partner.

These advantages and disadvantages are only summarized for your reference. A good Qigong masseur should practice both self-massage and mutual massage with a partner. A high level of Qigong massage can be achieved only through a lot of practice. Practice is the best way to accumulate experience.

6-2. Self-Massage

In this section we will introduce the various ways of using the hands to massage the body and smooth out the Qi circulation. The methods introduced in this and the next section are mainly used for maintaining health, improving the functioning of the body, and slowing down the aging process.

Generally speaking, whether you are massaging yourself or a partner, you follow the same routine. That is, when you are massaging for relaxation and to improve Qi and blood circulation you want to lead the Qi from the center out to the limbs, and from the top of the head down to the bottom of the feet. You therefore begin your massage with the head and neck.

The head is the center of your entire being. When you massage your head, you are starting to relax your mental body, which has to relax before your physical body can start to relax. Massaging the head also improves Qi and blood circulation there, which keeps the eyes and ears healthy. Vision and hearing are usually the first senses to start deteriorating as you age. This can be avoided or postponed by leading Qi to the head to nourish these organs. The first and crucial step in this is loosening up the neck, which is the passageway for the Qi and blood.

Once you have massaged your head and neck, you massage your chest and lead the Qi downward to the stomach. After you have finished massaging your chest and abdomen, you massage your limbs to improve the Qi circulation between them and the trunk of your body.

Although you use the same massage pathways when you massage yourself as when you are massaging someone else, there are a few significant differences and disadvantages. For example, we already know that massaging the spine is more important than massaging the chest, therefore it should be done first. However, when you massage yourself, it is impossible for your hands to reach your own spine. In order to remedy this, many people learn how to move the spine to loosen it. This will be discussed in the section on self-massage through movement. Another example is that it is very difficult to massage your own hips and the backs of your own thighs, which are the junctions of the Qi and blood between the body and the legs.

Self-Massage
1.   Head and Neck:
First Path:

Use your middle fingers to massage the bridge of your nose with a circular motion about five times (Figure 6-1). Then rub the fingers upward to the center of your forehead. Finally, gently stroke your hands to the top of your head, down the back of your neck, and out to your sides (Figure 6-2). Do this five to ten times. This path smoothes out the superficial Qi and blood circulation on your head.

Second Path:

Again circle your middle fingers on the bridge of your nose about five times and rub them upward to your forehead. Then brush with your middle and index fingers to the sides of your forehead, circle the temples a few times, and brush down to the jaws and chin (Figure 6-3). When you do this movement you may place your thumbs on the jaw to steady your hands. Repeat the procedure five to ten times. This path improves Qi and blood circulation in your face.

Figure 6-1.

Figure 6-2.

Figure 6-3.

Figure 6-4.

Third Path:

Again start at the bridge of your nose. Circle your middle fingers on the bridge of your nose five times, and then use your index and middle fingers to gently circle your eyes about five times (Figure 6-4). Finally, rub to the sides of your eyes and downward to the jaw. You may again use your thumbs to stabilize the massaging fingers. Repeat the procedure about five to ten times. Then rub your hands together until they are warm, and gently place the bases of your palms on your eyes to nourish them with the Qi from the palms (Figure 6-5). This is called "ironing the eyes" (Tang Yan). This path improves the Qi and blood circulation around the eyes and slows the deterioration of the eyes.

Figure 6-5.

Figure 6-6.

Figure 6-7.

Figure 6-8.

Fourth Path:

Gently press your index fingers in front of your ears, and rub lightly up and around the ears and finally down to the sides of the neck (Figure 6-6). Do this about five times. Next, cover your ears tightly with your hands and move your hands in a circle five times in one direction, and then five times in the other direction (Figure 6-7); finally, press your ears with your palms and then release to pop the ears five times (Figure 6-8). This path keeps the ears functioning properly.

Figure 6-9.   Figure 6-10.

Fifth Path:

This path leads the Qi and blood downward from the back of the neck. When you massage this path, lean your head slightly backward to relax the muscles in the back of your neck. Starting at the base of your skull, press and push with your thumbs down along the neck muscles on both sides of the spine (Figure 6-9). Repeat ten times. Then use your right hand to grab and rub the back of your neck ten times, and do the same thing with your left hand (Figure 6-10). This loosens up the neck, and allows the Qi and blood to pass through the neck more smoothly. However, you also need to lead any excess Qi down out of your head so that it doesn't stagnate there. The procedure is very simple: simply grab and massage your shoulder muscles on both sides with your fingers (Figure 6-11).

After you have massaged your head, you may slowly and gently move your head in a small circle ten times in each direction to help the neck muscles relax even more (Figure 6-12). Do not tilt your head all the way back, because this puts too much stress on the discs between the vertebrae.

2.   Chest:
First Path:

Brush with both hands from the back of your neck to the upper chest, and then follow the centerline downward to your abdomen (Figure 6-13). When your hands are on the back of your neck, inhale deeply, and when they are moving downward in front of your chest, exhale deeply while at the same time relaxing inside your chest. Repeat ten times.

Figure 6-11.

Figure 6-12.

Figure 6-13.

Figure 6-14.

Second Path:

This path starts under your throat. First place both of your hands under your throat (Figure 6-14), inhale deeply while staying relaxed, then exhale and at the same time brush your hands over both sides of your chest down to the bottom of your ribs (Figure 6-15). Repeat five times.

Third Path:

First, use the second and middle fingers of your left hand to gently massage the area just above your right nipple for one minute (Figure 6-16). Then use the second and middle fingers of your right

Figure 6-15.

Figure 6-16.

Figure 6-17.

Figure 6-18.

hand to massage the area just above your left nipple. This will lead the kidney Qi and water upward to moisten your lungs.

Next, place both palms on the center of your upper chest, inhale deeply, and then exhale and gently expand your chest as you move your palms to the sides of your upper chest (Figure 6-17). This will spread the Qi and moisture which was led upward to the sides of the lungs. Repeat five times.

Finally, place your palms on your solar plexus while inhaling, and then exhale and gently expand your chest while moving your palms to the sides of the middle of your chest (Figure 6-18). Repeat five times.

Figure 6-19.   Figure 6-20.

Fourth Path:

Rub the upper right side of your chest with the fingers of your left hand in a circular motion, and gradually move the motion downward to your lower ribs (Figure 6-19). Repeat five times. The direction of your circling is very important. When your left hand is circling clockwise (from the point of view of someone looking at you from the front), you are leading the Qi downward, which will cool down your body. If you reverse the direction, you are leading the Qi upward to your head, which is not desirable. Repeat the same movements with your left palm another five times (Figure 6-20).

Finally, massage the left side of your chest with your right hand, first with your fingertips, and then with your palm. Make sure that your are now circling counterclockwise so that you are leading the Qi down the center of your body.

Fifth Path:

Use your right thumb and fingers to grab and rub the tendons in front of your left armpit (Figure 6-21). Continue the grabbing and rubbing downward to the area of the nipple, and then use your palm to smooth and lead Qi down from your armpit (Figure 6-22). Repeat the same procedure about five times, and then do the other side.

3. Stomach, Abdomen, and Lower Back:
First Path:

First, place both hands on your stomach, and circle to the left and downward, continuing up the right side to the center of your stomach (Figure 6-23). Circle from ten to thirty times. While circling your hands, your mind should be very calm and relaxed. The more you relax deeply into your body, the more you can lead the Qi inside, and the more benefit you will receive.

Figure 6-21.

Figure 6-22.

Figure 6-23.

Figure 6-24.

Second Path:

Place your hands on either side of the centerline of your body at the level of your diaphragm. Inhale and then exhale deeply, while at the same time brushing both hands downward to the groin area (Figure 6-24).

Third Path:

Gently grab the tendons on the side of your waist and rub them for a few minutes (Figure 6-25), then use your palms to push down to the front of your thighs (Figure 6-26).

Figure 6-25.

Figure 6-26.

Figure 6-27.

Figure 6-28.

Fourth Path:

Close your hands into fists, and place the thumb-sides over your kidneys (Figure 6-27). Circle your fists for a few minutes. In the wintertime, circle your fists in toward the spine and down, and in the summertime, reverse the direction. When you finish circling, use the back of your fists to lightly strike your kidneys, sacrum, and the top portion of your hips for a few minutes (Figure 6-28). This will bring the stagnant Qi to the surface of the skin. Finally, starting in the area of the kidneys, brush downward with your hands past your hips and down to the back of your thighs (Figure 6-29).

Figure 6-29.

Figure 6-30.

Figure 6-31.

Figure 6-32.

4. Legs:

Starting at your hip, use the base of your palms to rub and move from the hip joints down the front of your thighs to your knees (Figure 6-30). There are three main paths on the front of the thighs: the center and the two sides. Next, grab and rub the muscles on the top of the thighs, moving from the hips down to your knees on each of the three pathways (Figure 6-31).

Next, use the base or the edge of your palms to rub and move from your hips down the outside of the thighs (Figure 6-32), and from your groin down the inside of your legs to the knees (Figure 6-33). Then

Figure 6-33.

Figure 6-34.

Figure 6-35.

Figure 6-36.

grab and rub the muscles on the sides and back of your thighs (Figure 6-34). When you massage the inside of your thighs, it is better to use the right hand to massage the left thigh, and vice versa.

Next, use your thumb, second finger, and/or the middle finger (whichever is easier) to press and vibrate some of the acupuncture cavities in your thighs (Figure 6-35). You should refer to the last chapter for the locations of the cavities in the legs. This will stimulate the cavities and enhance the Qi circulation in the primary channels. When you stimulate the cavities, start on the hips and work downward. When you have finished, brush downward with your hands from your hips to your knees (Figure 6-36). Repeat ten times.

Figure 6-37.

Figure 6-38.

Figure 6-39.

Figure 6-40.

Next, massage your knees and calves. First, use the base or the edge of your palms to massage your knees (Figure 6-37). Then use the base or the edge of your palms to press and rub downward from your knees to your ankles (Figure 6-38). After this, grab and rub the calf muscles (Figure 6-39). Then, stimulate the cavities in the calves (Figure 6-40). Finally, use your hands to brush downward to lead the Qi to your feet (Figure 6-41).

5. Feet:

We known from Chinese medicine that the hands and feet are actually connected and closely related to the internal organs. Six

Figure 6-41.

Order of Chi Circulation

From	To	Channel	Name	Time Period
Top of Chest	Outside of Thumb	Hand *Taiyin*	Lung	3 to 5 A.M.
Tip of Index Finger	Side of Nose	Hand *Yangming*	Large Intestine	5 to 7 A.M.
Under the Eye	Second Toe	Foot *Yangming*	Stomach	7 to 9 A.M.
Big Toe	Top of Chest	Foot *Taiyin*	Spleen	9 to 11 A.M.
Armpit	Little Finger	Hand *Shaoyin*	Heart	11 to 1 P.M.
Little Finger	Front of Ear	Hand *Taiyang*	Small Intestine	1 to 3 P.M.
Inner Corner of Eye	Little Toe	Foot *Taiyang*	Bladder	3 to 5 P.M.
Little Toe	Collarbone	Foot *Shaoyin*	Kidney	5 to 7 P.M.
Chest	Middle Finger	Hand *Jueyin*	Pericardium	7 to 9 P.M.
Ring Finger	Outside of Eyebrow	Hand *Shaoyang*	Triple Burner	9 to 11 P.M.
Outside Corner of the Eye	Fourth Toe	Foot *Shaoyang*	Gall Bladder	11 to 1 A.M.
Outside of Big Toe	Side of Nipple	Foot *Jueyin*	Liver	1 to 3 A.M.

Table 6-1. Qi circulation in the twelve primary channels.

primary Qi channels end in the fingers, and six in the toes (Table 6-1). There are many other zones on the hands and feet which are related to internal organs or even other parts of the body (Figure 6-42). Stimulating these channels and zones can improve the functioning of the related organs or parts of the body. This kind of stimula-

Right   Left

1. Pineal
2. Throat
3. Thyroid
4. Pituitary
5. Stomach
6. Hip and Knee
7. Gall Bladder
8. Lungs
9. Kidney
10. Sigmoid Colon
11. Transverse Colon
12. Descending Colon
13. Ascending Colon
14. Shoulder
15. Solar Plexus

16. Ear
17. Eye
18. Liver
19. Bladder
20. Adrenal
21. Appendix
22. Pancreas
23. Sciatic Nerve
24. Rectum
25. Small Intestine
26. Heart
27. Sinuses
28. Bronchial
29. Spleen
30. Thymus

Sciatic Nerve
Prostate
Kidneys
Illeocecal valve (r)
Sigmoid Colon (l)
Ovaries, Testes
Pelvic Area
Lymphatics

Lymphatics
Sciatic Nerve
Prostate
Bladder
Womb, Penis
Prostate
Pelvic Area
Rectum
Lower Lumbar

Figure 6-42. Massage zones for foot reflexology.

tion of the hands and feet is now commonly called "reflexology." We recommend that, when you finish the following general hand and foot massage, you devote some time to zone reflexology.

To massage your feet, first hold your foot and move it in a circle about twenty times in each direction (Figure 6-43). Then rub every portion of your feet with your thumb, using the other four fingers to stabilize the thumb and help regulate the power. Start with the back of the feet and toes (Figure 6-44). Pay special attention to the spaces between the bones. Next, press your thumb into the gaps between the bones, and drag or push from the ankle to the base of the toes (Figure 6-45). This will stimulate deep inside the foot. It will also remove any Qi and blood stagnation between the bones, which can interfere with the functioning of the foot, and even cause arthritis.

Figure 6-43.

Figure 6-44.

Figure 6-46.

Figure 6-45.

Repeat the massage on the bottoms of the feet (Figure 6-46), then press in with the thumbs between the bones and press or drag from the heel to the toes (Figure 6-47). Finally, grab the last section of each toe and gently pull and shake it (Figure 6-48).

After you have massaged your feet, stimulate the zones of the feet (Figure 6-42). To do this, press your thumb on each zone and rub in a circle.

6. Testicles:

Massaging the testicles increases the production of hormones. According to Chinese Muscle/Tendon Changing and Marrow/Brain

Figure 6-47.

Figure 6-48.

Washing Qigong (Yi Jin Jing and Xi Sui Jing), massaging the testicles correctly will increase hormone production and increase the amount of Qi led upward to the brain. Other effects are increasing the amount of Qi stored in the body and strengthening the immune system. There are many ways to massage the testicles. For example, you may hold the testicles gently between your palms and move your hands in a circle. You may also simply hold them in your hand and gently press and rub them. This subject is discussed in more detail in the YMAA book "Muscle/Tendon Changing and Marrow/Brain Washing Chi Kung."

7. Arms:

After you have finished massaging your legs, you finally massage your arms and hands. When you massage your arms, start with the muscles and tendons between the neck and the shoulders. Use the grabbing techniques to grab the muscles and rub around (Figure 6-49). Gradually move from your shoulders down to your hands to loosen up the muscles in your arms (Figure 6-50). Then use your thumb and your index and/or middle finger (depending on which is easier) to press and vibrate some of the acupuncture cavities in your arms (Figure 6-51). This will stimulate the cavities and enhance the Qi circulation in the primary channels. Please refer to the previous chapter for the locations of the cavities in the arms. When you stimulate the cavities, start at your shoulders and work downward. Repeat several times. After you finish the cavity press, brush downward with a hand from your shoulder to your hand (Figure 6-52). Repeat ten times.

8. Hands:

First, use your thumb to rub every portion of your wrist, hand, and fingers, starting on the back of the hand. Use the other four

Figure 6-49.

Figure 6-50.

Figure 6-51.

Figure 6-52.

fingers to stabilize your thumb and help to regulate the power (Figure 6-53). Pay special attention to the spaces between the bones. Next, press your thumb into the spaces between the bones in the hand, and drag or push from your wrist to the base of the fingers (Figure 6-54). This will help to stimulate the deeper places in your hand, and remove any Qi and blood stagnation between the bones which can hinder the functioning of the hands or even cause arthritis.

Repeat the rubbing massage on the palm side of your hand (Figure 6-55), and press in while dragging or pushing from your wrist to the base of the fingers (Figure 6-56).

Figure 6-53.

Figure 6-54.

Figure 6-55.

Figure 6-56.

Grab one finger at a time and pull lightly, letting the finger slip out of your grasp (Figure 6-57). Do each finger three times. This will lead the Qi to the fingertips. Finally, grab the last section of each finger and gently pull and shake it a few times (Figure 6-58).

When you have finished one hand, repeat the same process on the other one, then stimulate the zones mentioned earlier (Figure 6-59). To do this, simply press on the zone with your thumb and rub in a circle. Again, use the other four fingers to stabilize the thumb and control the power.

Figure 6-57.   Figure 6-58.

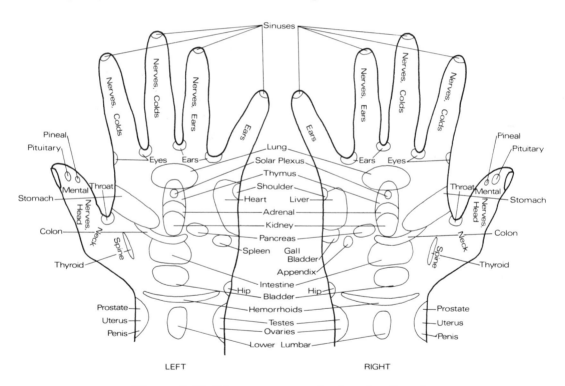

Figure 6-59. Massage zones for hand reflexology.

6-3. Self-Massage of the Internal Organs

In this section we would like to introduce two types of Qigong massage which are commonly used to improve Qi circulation around the internal organs. The first type of massage is for improving the Qi circulation around the internal organs by massaging either directly over the organs or on acupuncture cavities which are connected to

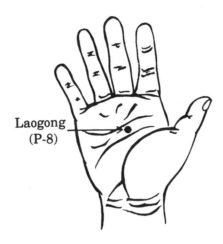

Figure 6-60. The Langong cavity.

the organs. The second type of practice is massaging the internal organs by moving the muscles inside the torso.

Your internal organs are the foundation of your health. Most deaths are due to malfunction or failure of the internal organs. In order to be healthy and avoid degeneration, your organs need to have the correct amount of Qi circulating smoothly through them. The internal organs manage the energy in our bodies, and carry out a variety of physical processes. When any organ starts to malfunction, the Qi circulation in the body will be disrupted, and the production of hormones will be affected. This state can result in a variety of disorders. Therefore, to maintain your health, you must first learn how to maintain the healthy functioning of your internal organs. To reach this goal, you have to learn how to keep the Qi and blood circulating smoothly in your organs.

Using the hands to massage the internal organs is a natural human instinct, and we do it whenever we feel pain or Qi stagnation in or near an organ. For example, if you have diarrhea and feel pain in your abdomen, you naturally massage yourself with your hands, and if you overeat, you automatically stroke or rub your stomach with your palms to ease the pain.

There are two methods of using the hands to massage the internal organs. The first method uses gentle rubbing to loosen and relax the muscles around the internal organs. In the second method, the hands are placed on the afflicted area, and Qi is released from the centers of the palms to remove Qi and blood stagnation around the internal organs. As you can probably guess, in the second method the Qi does the actual healing.

We mentioned earlier that in the center of each palm is a cavity or gate called the "Laogong" (Figure 6-60) which is used to regulate the Qi of the heart whenever the Qi flow is too strong. Unless you are sick, the Qi in the heart is normally more positive than is necessary, especially in the summertime. When you are excited or nervous, even more Qi accumulates around the heart. When this happens, the centers of your palms will feel warm and will often sweat.

Since the Qi in the center of the palm is always strong, you can use this Qi to help stagnant Qi in an organ to flow smoothly. Chinese physicians and Qigong practitioners have developed a number of ways of using the hands to improve the Qi circulation in the internal organs. In this section we will first introduce a few common methods for using the hands to massage the internal organs, and then we will explain how to use body movements to attain the same goal. These techniques can be practiced easily by anyone.

Massaging your Internal Organs with your Hands

Some of the techniques for massaging your internal organs are similar or identical to those discussed previously for massaging the waist. Since keeping the internal organs functioning properly is a goal shared by both general self-massage and self-massage of the organs, they both follow the same theory and use the same or similar techniques. However, regulating the Qi in the internal organs requires that the mind be in a more meditative and concentrated state so that you can reach deeply inside your body. You also need to build up your Qi so that it will be stronger and more penetrating. This takes more time than when you are only giving yourself a general self-massage.

We recommend that you compare the theory and techniques discussed in this section with those introduced in the previous one. This will give you a deeper understanding of the techniques.

1.   Large and Small Intestines:

To massage your abdomen and regulate the Qi circulation in your large and small intestines, place one hand on top of the other on your lower abdomen. If you are right-handed, it is better if you place your right hand on the bottom and the left hand on the top, and if you are left-handed, place your left hand on the bottom. The reason for this is quite simple: the Qi is strongest in the hand you use most often, and it is easier for you to lead the Qi from it.

When you massage your abdomen, it is best if you lie down so that your lower body is relaxed and the Qi can circulate more easily and smoothly. Hold your hand lightly against the skin and gently circle your hands clockwise, which is the direction of movement within the large intestine (Figure 6-61). Circling in the other direction would hinder the natural movements of peristalsis. Massage until you feel warm and comfortable deep inside your body.

As you massage, your breathing should be relaxed, deep, and comfortable. Place your mind a few inches under your palms. The mind will then be able to lead the Qi inward to smooth out Qi and blood stagnation.

Figure 6-61.   Figure 6-62.

2.   Liver, Stomach, Spleen, and Gall Bladder:

In Qigong massage for the internal organs, the liver, stomach, spleen, and gall bladder are usually included in the same techniques because they are all located in the middle of the front of the body. Maintaining healthy Qi circulation in an organ requires not only that the circulation in the organ itself be smooth, but also that the circulation between the organs be smooth. Therefore, when you massage these four internal organs, you should treat them as one instead of four.

Hold your hands as you did when massaging the lower abdomen, only now place them above the navel. Experience has shown that clockwise is again more effective than counterclockwise (Figure 6-62). It is also easiest to do this massage when you are lying down. Massage until you feel warm inside.

3.   Kidneys:

Chinese medicine considers the kidneys one of the most important internal organs. The kidneys affect how the other organs function, so almost all forms of Qigong place heavy emphasis on keeping them healthy.

To massage your own kidneys, close your hands into fists and place the thumb/index finger sides on your kidneys. Gently circle both fists until the kidneys are warm. In the summer, when your kidneys are normally too Yang, it is desirable to dissipate some of the Qi. This can be done by circling your right hand clockwise and your left hand counterclockwise (Figure 6-63). This leads the Qi to the sides of your body. However, when you massage your kidneys in the wintertime, when the kidney Qi is normally deficient, then you should reverse the direction and lead the Qi to the center of your back to nourish the kidneys. As usual, the breathing and the mind are important keys to successful practice.

There are other methods of improving the Qi circulation in the kidneys. The most common of which is to massage the bottoms of

Figure 6-63.

Figure 6-64. The Yongquan cavity.

your feet. There is a Qi gate in the front center of each sole which is called "Yongquan" (Gushing Spring)(Figure 6-64). Massaging these two cavities will stimulate the Qi circulation in the kidneys and help to regulate them (Figure 6-65).

4. Lungs:

According to the five elements theory, the lungs belong to Metal while the heart belongs to Fire. According to this theory, the Metal lungs can be used to regulate the heart Fire just as metal can absorb heat. If you pay attention carefully you will notice that when you feel heat around your heart because of excitement, you will normally thrust out your chest and greatly expand your lungs while inhaling. Doing this a few times reduces the pressure and the feeling of heat in the heart.

To do Qigong massage for your lungs, place both hands on the center of your chest just above the solar plexus (Figure 6-66). Inhale deeply, and then exhale while lightly pushing both hands to the sides (Figure 6-67). Do this until your lungs feel relaxed and comfortable. This massage is also good for the heart.

5. Heart:

Qigong teachers do not normally encourage students to massage their own hearts unless they are fairly advanced in skill. The heart is the most vital organ, and if you mistreat it you are in big trouble.

When you massage your heart, unlike all the other internal organs, you cannot place your mind on it. If you do place your mind on your heart you will lead more Qi to it and make it even more positive. You may have noticed that when your heart is beating fast after exercising, if you pay attention to your heartbeat it will start beating even faster. A person who is prone to heart attacks can pos-

Figure 6-65.

Figure 6-66.

Figure 6-67.

Figure 6-68.

sibly bring one on by paying too much attention to his heart. If your heart is beating too hard, the best thing is to pay attention to your lungs and breathe deeply and gently. After only a few breaths your heart will slow down and regain its regular pace.

Therefore, when you massage your heart, your mind should not be on your heart. Instead, keep your mind on the movement of your hands. To massage your heart, place your right hand over your heart at least three inches above your chest. Move your hand in a small clockwise circle, and gradually increase the size of the circle. This takes the Qi in the heart and spreads it out around the chest. Finally, lead the Qi past the liver and down the right leg (Figure 6-68).

Massaging the Internal Organs with Movement

In this section we will introduce methods for massaging the internal organs through body movements both when you are standing and also when you are sitting. This type of massage has been practiced in China for more than one thousand years. The Eight Pieces of Brocade is a very well known set of exercises that exemplifies this type of massage. If you would like to learn more about The Eight Pieces of Brocade, please refer to the YMAA book of that title.

The internal organs are surrounded by muscles, but, except for some of the trunk muscles which we use constantly throughout the day, most of these muscles are ignored. According to Qigong theory, if you can bring your Yi (mind) to a muscle, you can lead Qi to energize it and move it. For example, if you decide you want to be able to wiggle your ears, if you keep trying, you will eventually be able to. It's the same with the internal muscles. This means that if you practice becoming very calm and bringing your attention deeper and deeper into the center of your body, you will soon be able to feel and sense the structure and condition of the inside of your body. Once this happens, you can use your mind to move the internal muscles and massage the internal organs.

The way to gain control of the muscles inside your body is to start using your trunk muscles to make the movements. After you have practiced for a while, your mind will be able to reach deeper and feel other muscles as well. Once you are able to feel these muscles, you will be able to move them. With a bit more practice you will be able to control them while keeping them relaxed, and the movements will become natural, easy, and comfortable. Remember that the muscles have to be relaxed before the organs can be relaxed and before the Qi can circulate smoothly.

In this sub-section we will introduce the beginning steps of internal organ massage through trunk movement. After you are able to do these exercises easily and smoothly, you should continue to lead your mind deeper and deeper into your body until you can sense your organs.

It is a good idea to loosen up your trunk before starting these massaging movements. This will let you move more naturally and comfortably. The following stretching and warming up exercises can be used for both standing and sitting internal organ massage.

Loosening the Trunk Muscles:
The trunk is the center of the whole body, and it contains the muscles which control the trunk and also surround the internal organs. When the trunk muscles are tense, the whole body will be tense and the internal organs will be compressed. This causes stagnation of the Qi circulation in the body and especially in the organs. For this reason, the trunk muscles should be stretched and loosened up before any moving Qigong practice.

First, interlock your fingers and lift your hands up over your head while imagining that you are pushing upward with your hands and pushing downward with your feet (Figure 6-69). Do not tense your muscles, because this will constrict your body and prevent you from stretching. If you do this stretch correctly, you will feel the

Figure 6-69.   Figure 6-70.

muscles in your waist area tensing slightly because they are being pulled simultaneously from the top and the bottom.

Next, use your mind to relax even more, and stretch out a little bit more. After you have stretched for about ten seconds, turn your upper body to one side to twist the trunk muscles (Figure 6-70). Stay to the side for three to five seconds, turn your body to face forward and then turn to the other side. Stay there for three to five seconds. Repeat the upper body twisting three times, then tilt your upper body to the side and stay there for about three seconds (Figure 6-71), then tilt to the other side. Next, bend forward and touch your hands to the floor (Figure 6-72) and stay there for three to five seconds. Finally, squat down with your feet flat on the floor to stretch your ankles (Figure 6-73), and then lift your heels up to stretch the toes (Figure 6-74). Repeat the entire process ten times. After you finish, the inside of your body should feel very comfortable and warm.

The torso is supported by the spine and the trunk muscles. Once you have stretched your trunk muscles, you can loosen up the torso. This also moves the muscles inside your body around, which moves and relaxes your internal organs. This, in turn, makes it possible for the Qi to circulate smoothly inside your body.

Massaging the Internal Organs While Standing

a. Massaging the Large Intestine, Small Intestine, Urinary Bladder, and Kidneys:

This exercise helps you to regain conscious control of the muscles in your abdomen. There are four major benefits to this abdominal

Figure 6-71.

Figure 6-72.

Figure 6-73.

Figure 6-74.

exercise. First, when your Lower Dan Tian area is loose, the Qi can flow in and out easily. The Lower Dan Tian is the main residence of your Original Qi. The Qi in your Dan Tian can be led easily only when your abdomen is loose and relaxed. Second, when the abdominal area is loose, the Qi circulation in the large and small intestines will be smooth, and they will be able to absorb nutrients and eliminate waste efficiently. If your body does not eliminate effectively, the absorption of nutrients will be hindered, and you may become sick. Third, when the abdominal area is loose, the Qi in the kidneys will circulate smoothly and the Original Essence stored there can be converted more efficiently into Qi. In addition, when the kidney area is loosened, the kidney Qi can be led downward and upward to nourish the entire body. Fourth, these exercises eliminate Qi stagnation in the lower back, healing and preventing lower back pain.

To practice this exercise, stand with your feet a comfortable distance apart and your knees slightly bent. As you get more used to this exercise and your legs become stronger, bend your knees a little bit more. Without moving your thighs or upper body, use the waist muscles to move the abdomen around in a horizontal circle (Figure 6-75). Circle in one direction about ten times, and then in the other direction about ten times. If you hold one hand over your Lower Dan Tian and the other on your sacrum, you may be able to focus your attention better on the area you want to control.

In the beginning, you may have difficulty making your body move the way you want it to, but if you keep practicing you will quickly learn how to do it. Once you can do the movement comfortably, make the circles larger and larger. Naturally, this will cause the muscles to tense somewhat and inhibit the Qi flow, but the more you practice the sooner you will be able to relax again. After you have practiced for a while and can control your waist muscles easily, start making the circles smaller, and also start using your Yi to lead the Qi from the Dan Tian to move in these circles. The final goal is to have only a slight physical movement, but a strong movement of Qi.

When you practice, concentrate your mind on your abdomen and inhale and exhale deeply and smoothly. Remember that breathing deep does not mean breathing heavily. When you breathe deep, keep the muscles controlling the lungs and diaphragm relaxed. Inhale to lead the Qi into the center of the body and exhale to lead the Qi out from the skin.

b. Massaging the Stomach, Liver, Spleen, Gall Bladder, and Kidneys:

Beneath your diaphragm is your stomach, on its right are your liver and gall bladder, on its left is your spleen, and in the back are the kidneys. Once you can comfortably do the movement in your lower abdomen, change the movement from horizontal to vertical, and extend it up to your diaphragm. The easiest way to loosen the area around the diaphragm is to use a wave-like motion between the perineum and the diaphragm (Figure 6-76). You may find it helpful when you practice this to place one hand on your Lower Dan Tian and your other hand above it with the thumb on the solar plexus. Use a forward and backward wave-like motion, flowing up to the diaphragm and down to the perineum and back. While you do this,

Figure 6-75.   Figure 6-76.

inhale deeply when the motion is starting at the perineum and exhale as it reaches the diaphragm. Practice ten times.

Next, continue the movement while turning your body slowly to one side and then to the other (Figure 6-77). This will slightly tense the muscles on one side and loosen them on the other, which will massage the internal organs. Repeat ten times.

This exercise loosens the muscles around the stomach, liver, gall bladder, spleen, and kidneys, and therefore improves the Qi circulation there. It also trains you in using your mind to lead Qi from your Lower Dan Tian upward to the solar plexus area.

c.   Massaging the Lungs and Heart:

This exercise loosens up the chest and helps to regulate and improve the Qi circulation in the lungs. According to the theory of the five phases in Chinese medicine, the lungs belong to the element Metal while the heart belongs to the element Fire. Metal is able to cool down Fire, and the lungs are able to regulate the Qi of the heart. The heart is the most vital organ, and its condition is closely related to our life and death. If there is too much Qi in the heart (when it is too Yang), you speed up its degeneration and become prone to heart attacks. For this reason, Qigong places great emphasis on using the lungs to regulate the Qi in the heart. If we know how to relax the lungs and keep the Qi circulating in them smoothly, they will be able to regulate the heart more efficiently.

After loosening up the center portion of your body, extend the movement up to your chest. The wave-like movement starts in the abdomen, moves through the stomach and up to the chest. You

Figure 6-77.

Figure 6-78.

may find it easier to feel the movement if you hold one hand on your abdomen and the other lightly touching your chest (Figure 6-78). After you have done the movement ten times, extend the movement to your shoulders (Figure 6-79). Inhale when you move your shoulders backward and exhale when you move them forward. The inhalation and exhalation should be as deep as comfortably possible, and the entire chest should be very loose. Repeat the motion ten times.

Massaging the Internal Organs While Sitting

The theory of self-massage of the internal organs with movement is the same whether you are standing or sitting. The only difference is that when you are sitting, the internal organs in the lower part of body such as the urinary bladder, large intestine, and small intestine cannot be massaged as easily as when you are standing.

Self-massage of the organs with movement is not as easy or convenient to do when you are sitting, but it can still be very valuable for people who have difficulty standing. As a matter of fact, since ancient times many Chinese have practiced these movements right after awakening in the morning. "The Sitting Eight Pieces of Brocade" is a popular set of exercises that was created for this purpose. If you are interested in this set, you may refer to the YMAA publication: "The Eight Pieces of Brocade."

I believe that many people today will find the sitting self-massage of the organs to be more useful than the standing exercises.

Figure 6-79.   Figure 6-80.

Many jobs require long hours sitting in front of a computer terminal
or in a car, and uncomfortable feelings in the internal organs are a
common experience. The sitting exercises are just the thing to
relieve tension in the internal organs, improve Qi and blood circulation, and keep the organs healthy.

Loosening Up the Spine and Trunk Muscles

Before you massage your internal organs with movement, you
should first loosen up your spine and trunk muscles. First, starting
at your sacrum, move your spine in a wave-like motion upward to
your neck (Figure 6-80). Keep your body as relaxed as possible,
especially your trunk muscles. Repeat about ten times. Then, continue the same motion while slowly turning your body to the sides
(Figure 6-81). Finally, turn your body slowly to one side and then
the other as much as you can to stretch the trunk muscles (Figure 6-
82). Do this about five times to each side.

a. Massaging the Large and Small Intestines and the Urinary Bladder:

First learn how to move the muscles in your lower abdomen.
Inhale deeply and slowly while expanding your abdomen and gently
pushing your anus and Huiyin cavity out (Figure 6-83). Then,
exhale deeply and slowly while withdrawing your abdomen and
gently pulling in your anus and Huiyin cavity. Keep your mind calm
and natural, and your body centered and relaxed. Repeat about ten
to twenty times. This up and down movement massages the organs
in the lower abdomen.

Figure 6-81.

Figure 6-82.

Figure 6-83.

Figure 6-84.

Interlock your fingers and place them behind your head. Continue inhaling and exhaling deeply. As you exhale, slowly bend your body forward, and as you inhale, straighten up (Figure 6-84). Repeat ten times.

Finally, place your hands on your knees and repeat the same movements (Figure 6-85). With your hands on your knees your

Figure 6-85.

Figure 6-86.

Figure 6-87.

Figure 6-88.

trunk muscles can relax more, and the movements can reach deeper into the body.

b.   Massaging the Liver, Gall Bladder, Stomach, Spleen, and Kidneys:

Figure 6-89.   Figure 6-90.

As you did in the preceding section, bend forward and straighten up in coordination with your breathing. Now, however, keep your attention on the middle of your body, at the level of your lower ribs, rather than on your stomach. This will focus the movement there, and massage the liver and other organs there.

Next, inhale deeply, and raise your left hand and press down your right hand as you exhale (Figure 6-86). As you inhale, lower your left arm. Then raise your right hand and press down your left hand as you you exhale, and lower it as your inhale. Remember that deep and relaxed breathing is the key to massaging the internal organs in the middle of the body. When you breathe correctly, your diaphragm moves up and down, alternately applying and releasing pressure on the organs. Raise and lower each arm at least five times.

Next, continue raising and lowering your arms in coordination with your breathing, only now start turning your body from side to side (Figure 6-87). As you raise your right hand, turn to your left, and as you raise your left hand, turn to your right. Repeat ten times.

When you are through, still your mind and breathe deeply for a few minutes.

c. **Massaging the Lungs and Heart:**
Continue normal abdominal breathing. As you inhale, gently circle your shoulders to the rear, and as you exhale, circle them forward (Figure 6-88). Repeat the motion ten times, and then do ten more repetitions circling in the other direction.

Finally, raise your hands in front of your chest while inhaling (Figure 6-89), and circle them forward, to the sides, and then down to your waist as you exhale (Figure 6-90). Repeat ten times.

We have introduced you to only a few of the many techniques for massaging your internal organs. We hope that it is enough to serve you as an adequate introduction. Once you understand the theory and have accumulated some experience, you should be able to discover other movements and techniques which are also beneficial.

Chapter 7
Conclusion

Now that you have read this book, the next step is to practice self-massage by yourself and to also find a partner with whom you can practice general massage. Always remember that knowledge is only the Yin side of study. To become proficient you also need to manifest the Yang side through action.

During the course of your study, you should refer to the many other books about massage that are available. The more you read and study, the better you will be, and the more your knowledge will increase. If you can gather the opinions of many authors and learn through them the correct path, then you will surely be a wise practitioner.

You should also understand that this book is only the first part of an entire series of Chinese Qigong massage. The massage in this book is limited to maintaining health. If, after finishing this book, you wish to go on and enter the field of Qigong massage for healing, you should read the next volume in this series.

Appendix A
Glossary of Chinese Terms

An: 按

Press. A major technique of Chinese massage.

An Mo: 按摩

Literally: press rub. Together they mean massage.

Bai He: 白鶴

White Crane. A style of Chinese martial arts.

Baihui: 百會

Literally "hundred meetings." An important acupuncture cavity located on the top of the head. The Baihui cavity belongs to the Governing Vessel. Baihui is called "Tianlingai" in the Chinese martial arts and "Niwangong" in Daoist society.

Bagua: 八卦

Literally: Eight Divinations. Also called the Eight Trigrams. In Chinese philosophy, the eight basic variations; shown in the Yi Jing as groups of single and broken lines.

Bian Shi: 砭石

Stone Probe. Bian Shi were used to stimulate acupuncture cavities in the treatment of illnesses during the Yellow Emperor era (2690-2590 B.C.) before metal needles became available.

Cao Jie: 操接

Cao means "to operate" and Jie means "to connect." Cao Jie is a common name for bone connection in Fujian and Taiwan. Cao Jie is commonly done by martial artists.

Changquan (Chang Chuan): 長拳

Chang means long, and Quan means fist, style, or sequence. A style of Northern Chinese Gongfu which specializes in kicking and long range fighting. Changquan has also been used to refer to Taijiquan.

Chong Mai: 衝脈

Thrusting Vessel. One of the eight extraordinary vessels.

Dai Mai: 帶脈

Girdle Vessel. One of the eight extraordinary vessels.

Dan Tian: 丹田

Literally: Field of Elixir. Locations in the body which are able to store and generate Qi (elixir) in the body. The Upper, Middle, and Lower Dan Tian are located respectively between the eyebrows, at the solar plexus, and a few inches below the navel.

Dao (Tao): 道

The way. The "natural" way of everything.

Di: 地

The Earth. Earth, Heaven (Tian), and Man (Ren) are the "Three Natural Powers" (San Cai).

Di Li Shi: 地理師

Di Li means geomancy and Shi means teacher. Therefore Di Li Shi means a teacher or master who analyzes geographic locations according to formulas in the Yi Jing (Book of Change) and the energy distributions in the Earth.

Dian Qi: 電氣

Dian means electricity, and so Dian Qi means "electrical energy" (electricity). In China, a word is often placed before "Qi" to identify the different kinds of energy.

Dian Xue: 點穴

Dian means "to point and exert pressure" and Xue means "the cavities." Dian Xue refers to those Qin Na techniques which specialize in attacking acupuncture cavities to immobilize or kill an opponent.

Die Da: 跌打

Die means "fallen" and Da means "struck." Die Da is one of a number of names for the methods used by martial artists to treat injuries.

Du Mai: 督脉

Usually translated Governing Vessel. One of the eight extraordinary vessels.

Feng Shui Shi: 風水師

Literally: wind water teacher. Teacher or master of geomancy. Geomancy is the art or science of analyzing the natural energy relationships in a location, especially the interrelationships between "wind" and "water," hence the name. Also called Di Li Shi.

Feng Yang Men: 鳳陽門

Phoenix Sun Style. A Daoist martial art and meditation system which also specializes in Qigong massage.

Fu: 腑

The bowels. The Yang organs: the Gall Bladder, Small Intestine, Large Intestine, Stomach, Bladder, and Triple Burner.

Fujian: 福建

A province located in the southeast corner of China.

Hukou: 虎口

Tiger mouth. An acupuncture cavity located between the bases of the thumb and the second finger. Tiger mouth is called "Hegu" in Chinese medicine.

Gongfu (Kung Fu): 功夫

Literally: energy-time. Any study, learning, or practice which requires a lot of patience, energy, and time to complete. Since practicing Chinese martial arts requires a great deal of time and energy, Chinese martial arts are commonly called Gongfu.

Gu Zhen: 骨針

Bone needle. An acupuncture needle made from animal bone. Gu Zhen were used for acupuncture before metal needles were introduced.

Gui Qi: 鬼氣

The Qi residue of a dead person. It is believed by the Chinese Buddhists and Daoists that this Qi residue is a so called ghost.

Guoshu: 國術

Literally: national techniques. Another name for Chinese martial arts. First used by President Chiang Kai-Shek in 1926 at the founding of the Nanking Central Guoshu Institute.

Hegu: 合谷

An acupuncture cavity located between the bases of the thumb and the second finger. Hegu is also commonly called "Hukou."

Hsing Yi Chuan (Xingyiquan): 形意拳

Literally: Shape-mind Fist. An internal style of Gongfu in which the mind or thinking determines the shape or movement of the body. Creation of the style is attributed to Marshal Yue Fei.

Huo Qi: 活氣

Vital Qi. The Qi in living things.

Jia Gu Wen: 甲骨文

Oracle-Bone Scripture. Earliest evidence of the Chinese use of the written word. Found on pieces of turtle shell and animal bone from the Shang dynasty (1766-1154 B.C.). Most of the information recorded was of are ligius nature.

Jie: 結

Knots. Usually located on the junctions of blood or Qi vessels.

Jing: 經

Channel. Sometimes translated meridian. Refers to the twelve organ-related "rivers" which circulate Qi throughout the body.

Jing: 精

Essence. The most refined part of anything.

Jing: 勁

A power in Chinese martial arts which is derived from muscles which have been energized by Qi to their maximum potential.

Jing Qi: 精氣

Essence Qi. The Qi which has been converted from Original Essence.

Jueyin: 厥陰

Absolute Yin. One of the six classifications in Chinese acupuncture of the Qi state in the Qi primary channels.

Kan: 坎

A phase of the eight trigrams representing water.

Kan-Li: 坎離

Water-fire. The methods of adjusting the body's Yin and Yang condition.

Lao Zi: 老子

The creator of Daoism, also called Li Er.

Li: 離

A phase of the Bagua, Li represents fire.

Luo: 絡

The small Qi channels which branch out from the primary Qi channels and are connected to the skin and to the bone marrow.

Mi Zong: 密宗

Secret style. A Tibetan Buddhist society which specializes in meditation and martial arts.

Mo: 摩

Rub. A major technique of Chinese Qigong massage.

Na: 拿

Grab. A major technique of Chinese Tui Na Qigong massage.

Nan Jing: 難經

Difficulty classic. The name of an ancient Chinese medical book written by Qin Yue-Ren during the Zhou dynasty (1122-255 B.C.).

Nei Dan: 內丹

Literally: internal elixir. A form of Qigong in which Qi (the elixir) is built up in the body and spread out to the limbs.

Nei Jing: 內經

Internal classic. The name of the oldest Chinese medical book. It contains two major parts: Su Wen and Ling Shu.

Niwangong: 泥丸宮

A Daoist name for the cavity on the top of the head. It is also called "Tianlingai" in the Chinese martial arts and "Baihui" in Chinese medicine.

Pu Tong An Mo: 普通按摩

General massage. A category of Chinese Qigong massage.

Qi: 氣

The general definition of Qi is: universal energy, including heat, light, and electromagnetic energy. A narrower definition of Qi refers to the energy circulating in human or animal bodies.

Qi Hua Lun: 氣化論

Qi variation thesis. An ancient treatise which discusses the variations of Qi in the universe.

Qi Jing Ba Mai: 奇經八脈

Literally: strange channels odd vessels. Usually referred to as the eight extraordinary vessels, or simply as the vessels. Called odd or strange because they are not well understood and do not exist in pairs.

Qi Mai: 氣脈

Qi vessels. The eight vessels involved with transporting, storing, and regulating Qi.

Qi Shi: 氣勢

Shi means the way something looks or feels. Therefore: the feeling of Qi as it expresses itself.

Qi Xue: 氣血

Literally "Qi blood." According to Chinese medicine, Qi and

blood cannot be separated in our body, and so the two words are commonly used together.

Qian Long Men: 乾龍門

The name of a Daoist society.

Qiao: 蹻

The heel. Qiao is also a name for the Chinese massage technique which uses the feet.

Qiao Men: 窍門

The secret or tricky entrance. Qian Men is commonly used to refer to the key points which you need to know when entering into a new field of knowledge or practice.

Qigong (Chi Kung): 氣功

Gong means Gongfu (lit. energy-time). Therefore, Qigong means study, research, and/or practices related to Qi.

Qin Na (Chin Na): 擒拿

Literally, grab control. A type of Chinese Gongfu which emphasizes grabbing techniques to control the opponent's joints in conjunction with attacking certain acupuncture cavities.

Re Qi: 熱氣

Re means warmth or heat. Generally, Re Qi is used to represent heat. It is used sometimes to imply that a person or animal is still alive since the body is warm.

Ren: 人

Man or mankind.

Ren Mai: 任脉

Usually translated Conception Vessel. One of the eight extraordinary vessels.

Ren Qi: 人氣

Human Qi.

Ren Shi: 人事

Literally: human relations. Human events, activities, and relationships.

San Cai: 三才

Three powers. Heaven, Earth, and Man.

Shang Dan Tian: 上丹田

Upper Dan Tian. Located at the third eye, it is the residence of the Shen (spirit).

Shaolin: 少林

A Buddhist temple in Henan province, famous for its martial arts.

Shaoyang: 少陽

Lesser Yang. One of the six classifications in Chinese acupuncture of the Qi state of Qi primary channels.

Shaoyin: 少陰

Means "lesser Yin." One of the six classifications of the Qi state in Chinese acupuncture Qi primary channels.

Shen: 神

Spirit. According to Chinese Qigong, the Shen resides at the Upper Dan Tian (the third eye).

Shen Long: 神龍

Spiritual Dragon, a Daoist society.

Shi Zhen: 石針

Stone needle. Stone needles were used for acupuncture before metal needles were invented.

Si Qi: 死氣

Dead Qi. The Qi remaining in a dead body. Sometimes called ghost Qi (Gui Qi).

Su Wen: 素問

The first part of the the medical treatise Nei Jing. The second part is Ling Shu.

Suan Ming Shi: 算命師

Literally: calculate life teacher. A fortune teller who is able to calculate your future and destiny.

Taijiquan (Tai Chi Chuan): 太极拳

Great Ultimate Fist. A style of Chinese internal martial arts which emphasizes the cultivation of internal Qi. The creation of Taijiquan during the Chinese Song dynasty (960-1206 A.D.) is credited to Zhang San-Feng.

Taiyang: 太陽

Greater Yang. One of the six classifications in Chinese acupuncture of the Qi state of Qi primary channels.

Taiyin: 太陰

Greater Yin. One of the six classifications in Chinese acupuncture of the Qi state of Qi primary channels.

Taizuquan: 太祖拳

A style of Chinese martial arts which is said to have been created by Song Taizu, founder of the Song dynasty.

Tian: 天

Heaven or sky. In ancient China, people believed that heaven was the most powerful natural energy in this universe.

Tian Qi: 天氣

Heaven Qi. It is now commonly used to mean the weather, since weather is governed by heaven Qi.

Tian Shi: 天時

Heavenly timing. The repeated natural cycles generated by the heavens such as: seasons, months, days, and hours.

Tianlingai: 天靈蓋

Heavenly spiritual cover. A term used in the Chinese martial arts for the cavity on the top of the head. Tianlingai is also called "Niwangong" in Daoist society and "Baihui" in Chinese medicine.

Tui: 推

Push. A major technique in Chinese Tui Na Qigong massage.

Tui Na: 推拿

Literally: push grab. Tui Na is one of the traditional Chinese massage styles which specializes in using pushing and grabbing to adjust abnormal Qi circulation and cure sicknesses.

Wai Dan: 外丹

External elixir. External Qigong exercises in which a practitioner will build up his Qi in his limbs and then lead it into the center of the body for nourishment.

Wai Qi Liao Fa: 外氣療法

Wai Qi means "external Qi" and Liao Fa means "techniques for healing." Wai Qi Liao Fa is a Qigong healing method which uses Qi emitted by the healer.

Wei Qi: 衛氣

Protective Qi or Guardian Qi. The Qi at the surface of the body which generates a shield to protect the body from negative external influences such as colds.

Wu Xing: 五行

Five phases. Also called the five elements. Metal, wood, water, fire, and earth, representing the five phases of any process.

Wudang Mountain: 武當山

Located in Fubei province in China.

Wushu: 武術

Literally: martial techniques. A common name for the Chinese martial arts. Many other terms are used, including: Wuyi (martial arts), Wugong (martial Gongfu), Guoshu (national techniques), and Gongfu (energy-time). Because Wushu has been modified in mainland China over the past forty years into gymnastic martial performance, many traditional Chinese martial artist have given up this name in order to avoid confusing modern Wushu with traditional Wushu. Recently, mainland China has attempted to bring modern Wushu back toward its traditional training and practice.

Xi Sui Jing: 洗髓經

Literally: Washing Marrow Classic, usually translated Marrow Washing Classic. A Qigong training which specializes in leading Qi to the marrow to cleanse it. It is believed that Xi Sui Jing training is the key to longevity and reaching spiritual enlightenment.

Xia Dan Tian: 下丹田

Lower Dan Tian. Located in the lower abdomen, it is believed to be the residence of water Qi (Original Qi).

Xin: 心

Literally: Heart. Refers to the emotional mind.

Xingyiquan (Hsing Yi Chuan): 形意拳

Literally: Shape-mind Fist. An internal style of Gongfu in which the mind or thinking determines the shape or movement of the body. Creation of the style is attributed to Marshal Yue Fei.

Xue: 穴

Literally: cave or hole. An acupuncture cavity.

Yang: 陽

In Chinese philosophy, the active, positive, masculine polarity. In Chinese medicine, Yang means excessive, overactive, overheated. The Yang (or outer) organs are the Gall Bladder, Small Intestine, Large Intestine, Stomach, Bladder, and Triple Burner.

Yangming: 陽明

Yang brightness. One of the six classifications in Chinese acupuncture of the Qi state of Qi primary channels.

Yangqiao Mai: 陽蹻脉

Yang Heel Vessel. One of the eight extraordinary vessels.

Yangwei Mai: 陽維脉

Yang Linking Vessel. One of the eight extraordinary vessels.

Yi: 意

Mind. Specifically, the mind which is generated by clear thinking and judgement, and which is able to make you calm, peaceful, and wise.

Yi Jin Jing: 易筋經

Literally: changing muscle/tendon classic, usually called The Muscle/Tendon Changing Classic. Credited to Da Mo around 550 A. D., this work discusses Wai Dan Qigong training for strengthening the physical body.

Yi Jing: 易經

Book of Changes. A book of divination written during the Zhou dynasty (1122-255 B.C.).

Yin: 陰

In Chinese philosophy, the passive, negative, feminine polarity. In Chinese medicine, Yin means deficient. The Yin (internal) organs are the Heart, Lungs, Liver, Kidneys, Spleen, and Pericardium.

Yin Qi: 陰氣

The Qi state which is weaker than normal.

Yin Xu: 殷墟

A burial ground in An Yang, Henan province, used during the Shang dynasty (1766-1154 B.C.).

Ying Qi: 營氣

Managing Qi. The Qi which manages the functioning of the organs and the body.

Ying Zhua Men: 鷹爪門

Eagle claw style. A style of Chinese martial arts.

Yinqiao Mai: 陰蹻脉

Yin Heel Vessel. One of the eight extraordinary vessels.

Yinwei Mai: 陰維脉

Yang Linking Vessel. One of the eight extraordinary vessels.

Yuan Jing: 元精

Original Essence. The fundamental, original substance inherited from your parents, it is converted into Original Qi.

Zang: 臟

Viscera. The six Yin organs. Five of these are considered the core of the entire human system: the Liver, Heart, Spleen, Lungs, and Kidneys. Usually, when a discussion involves the channels and all the Organs, the Pericardium is added, otherwise it is treated as an adjunct of the Heart.

Zhen Shi: 箴石

Stone needle. Same as Shi Zhen.

Zheng Gu Ke: 正骨科

Align bone category. A medical training category in the Yuan dynasty (1206-1368 A.D.).

Zheng Qi: 正氣

Righteous Qi. When a person is righteous, it is said that he has righteous Qi, which evil Qi cannot overcome.

Zhong Dan Tian: 中丹田

Middle Dan Tian. Located in the area of the solar plexus, it is the residence of fire Qi.

Zhong Jiao: 中焦

Middle Triple Burner. The section of the Triple Burner which is located between the diaphragm and the navel.

Zhua Long: 抓龍

Zhua means "to grab," and Long means "dragon" and refers to the tendons and muscles. Zhua Long is a common name for general massage in Taiwan.

Appendix B
Translation of Chinese Terms

楊美玲 Mei-Ling Yang
氣功 Qigong
按摩 An Mo
推拿 Tui Na
點穴 Dian Xue
外氣療法 Wai Qi Liao Fa
普通按摩 Pu Tong An Mo
吳文慶 Wen-Ching Wu
楊俊敏 Yang Jwing-Ming
新竹縣 Xinzhu Xian
臺灣 Taiwan
武術 Wushu
功夫 Gongfu (Kung Fu)
少林 Shaolin
白鶴 Bai He
曾金灶 Cheng Gin-Gsao
太祖拳 Taizuquan
太祖 Taizu
金紹峰 Jin Shao-Feng
擒拿 Qin Na (Chin Na)
太极拳 Taijiquan (Tai Chi Chuan)
高濤 Kao Tao
李茂清 Li Mao-Ching
陳威伸 Wilson Chen
韓慶堂 Han Ching-Tan
張詳三 Chang Xiang-San
淡江學院 Tamkang College
長拳 Changquan (Chang Chuan)
國術 Guoshu

劲 Jing
形意拳 Hsing Yi Chuan (Xingyiquan)
連步拳 Lien Bu Chuan
功力拳 Gung Li Chuan
吳誠德 Wu Chengde
道 Dao (Tao)
拼音 Pinyin
氣 Qi

Chapter 1
陰 Yin
陽 Yang
氣功 Chi Kung (Qigong)
空氣 Kong Qi
三才 San Cai
天 Tian
地 Di
人 Ren
天氣 Tian Qi
電氣 Dian Qi
熱氣 Re Qi
人氣 Ren Qi
活氣 Huo Qi
死氣 Si Qi
鬼氣 Gui Qi
正氣 Zheng Qi
氣勢 Qi Shi
功 Gong
易經 Yi Jing
八卦 Bagua

氣化論	Qi Hua Lun	黃帝內經	Huang Di Nei Jing
天時	Tian Shi	素問	Su Wen
地理師	Di Li Shi	血氣形志篇	Xue Qi Xing Zhi Pian
風水師	Feng Shui Shi	經	Jing
人事	Ren Shi	絡	Luo
算命師	Suan Ming Shi	異法方宜論	Yi Fa Fang Yi Lun
抓龍	Zhua Long	蹻	Qiao
跌打	Die Da	葛洪	Ge Hong
正骨科	Zheng Gu Ke	時后救卒方	Shi Hou Jiu Zu Fang
明朝	Ming dynasty	人中	Renzhong
接骨科	Jie Gu Ke	抱朴子	Bao Pu Zi
福建	Fujian	隋朝	Sui dynasty
操接	Cao Jie	隋書百官志	Sui Shu Bai Guan Zhi
道士	Daoist	巢元方	Chao Yuan-Fang
易筋經	Yi Jin Jing	諸病源後論	Zhu Bing Yuan Hou Lun
洗髓經	Xi Sui Jing	唐朝	Tang dynasty
武當	Wudang	唐書職官志	Tang Shu Zhi Guan Zhi
夏朝	Xia dynasty	唐六典	Tang Liu Dian
石針	Shi Zhen	王燾	Wang Tao
砭石	Bian Shi	外臺秘要	Wai Tai Mi Yao
骨針	Gu Zhen	千金方	Qian Jin Fang
山海經	Shan Hai Jing	老子	Lao Zi
東山經	Dong Shan Jing	蘭道人	Lan Dao-Ren
高	Gao	仙授理傷續斷秘方	Xian Shou Li Shang Xu Duan Mi Fang
箴石	Zhen Shi	唐天寶	Tang Tian Bao
世郭璞	Shi Guo-Pu	經濟總論	Jing Ji Zong Lun
許慎	Xu Shen	儒門視事	Ru Men Shi Shi
説文解字	Shuo Wen Jie Zi	危亦林	Wei Yi-Lin
漢朝	Han dynasty	世醫得效方	Shi Yi De Xiao Fang
砭	Bian	元朝	Yuan dynasty
商朝	Shang dynasty	李仲南	Li Zhong-Nan
殷墟	Yin Xu	永類鈐方	Yong Lei Qian Fang
甲骨文	Jia Gu Wen	明朝	Ming dynasty
周朝	Zhou dynasty	朱橚	Zhu Su
禮記	Li Ji	普濟方，折傷門	Pu Ji Fang, Ze Shang Men
月令孟秋	Yue Ling Meng Qiu	王肯堂	Wang Ken-Tang
內經	Nei Jing	瘍醫準繩	Yang Yi Zhun Sheng
清朝	Qing dynasty	小兒按摩經	Xiao Er An Mo Jing
扁鵲	Bian Que	小兒推拿秘訣	Xiao Er Tui Na Mi Jue
子游	Zi You	楊繼洲	Yang Ji-Zhou
華陀	Hua Tuo	針灸大成	Zhen Jiu Da Cheng
張機作	Zhang Ji-Zuo	保嬰神術按摩經	Bao Ying Shen Shu
傷寒染病論	Shang Han Ran Bing Lun		
漢書藝文志	Han Shu Yi Wen Zhi		
歧伯	Qi Bo		
張仲景	Zhang Zhong-Jing		
金匱要略	Jin Kui Yao Lue		

An Mo Jing

胡埏壁 Hu Lian-Bi

小兒推拿方脉活嬰 Xiao Er Tui Na Fang
秘旨全書 Mai Huo Ying Mi Zhi
Quan Shu

周嶽甫 Zhou Yu-Fu
呈謙 Cheng Qian

醫宗金鑒 Yi Zong Jin Jian
正骨心法要旨 Zheng Gu Xin Fa Yao
Zhi

摸 Mo
接 Jie
端 Duan
提 Ti
推 Tui
拿 Na
按 An
摩 Mo

錢秀昌 Qian Xiu-Chang
傷科補要 Shang Ke Bu Yao
顧世澄 Gu Shi-Cheng
瘍醫大全 Yang Yi Da Quan
胡廷光 Hu Ting-Guang
傷科匯纂 Shang Ke Hui Cuan
越竹泉 Yue Zhu-Quan
傷科大成 Shang Ke Da Cheng
熊應雄 Xiong Ying-Xiong
推拿廣義 Tui Na Guang Yi
夏禹鑄 Xia Yu-Zhu
幼科鐵鏡 You Ke Tie Jing
駱潛庵 Luo Qian-An
幼科推拿秘術 You Ke Tui Na Mi Shu
鷹爪門 Ying Zhua Men
乾龍門 Qian Long Men
鳳陽門 Feng Yang Men
密宗 Mi Zong
神龍 Shen Long
雲斬 Yun Zhan
丁繼華 Ding Ji-Hua
蕭文忠 Xiao Wen-Zhong
李茂林 Li Mao-Lin

Chapter 2
膻中 Shanzhong
臟 Zang
腑 Fu
五行 Wu Xing
氣脉 Qi Mai

血 Xue
太陽 Taiyang
少陽 Shaoyang
陽明 Yangming
太陰 Taiyin
少陰 Shaoyin
厥陰 Jueyin
中焦 Zhong Jiao
元精 Yuan Jing
難經 Nan Jing
外丹 Wai Dan
內丹 Nei Dan
奇經八脉 Qi Jing Ba Mai
督脉 Du Mai
任脉 Ren Mai
衝脉 Chong Mai
帶脉 Dai Mai
陽蹻脉 Yangqiao Mai
陰蹻脉 Yinqiao Mai
陽維脉 Yangwei Mai
陰維脉 Yinwei Mai
營氣 Ying Qi
衛氣 Wei Qi
精氣 Jing Qi
坎離 Kan-Li
心 Xin
意 Yi
結 Jie
氣血 Qi Xue
窍門 Qiao Men
合谷 Hegu
虎口 Hukou
百會 Baihui
天靈蓋 Tianlingai
泥丸宮 Niwangong

Chapter 3
揉 Rou
摸 Mo
點打 Dian Da
敲 Qiao
震顫 Zhen Zhan
端 Duan
提 Ti
捏 Nie
頂 Ding
搖 Yao
拍 Pai

俞府 Shufu
氣戶 Qifu
中府 Zhongfu
鳩尾 Jiuwei
膺窗 Yinchuang
乳中 Ruzhong
乳根 Rugen
日月 Riyue
鼠蹊 Shuxi
急脉 Jimai
伏兔 Futu
舉臂 Jubi
肩内陵 Jianneiling
曲澤 Quze

Chapter 6
内臟按摩 Nei Zang An Mo

Chapter 7

Appendix A
蔣介石 Chiang Kai-Shek
南京中央國術館 Nanking Central
Guoshu Institute
岳飛 Yue Fei
李耳 Li Er
秦越人 Qin Yue-Ren
靈樞 Ling Shu
張三豐 Zhang San-Feng
宋太祖 Song Taizu
武藝 Wuyi
武功 Wugong

INDEX